THE INTERMITTENT FASTING JOURNEY FOR WOMEN

A COMPLETE BEGINNER'S GUIDE TO ACHIEVING ULTIMATE WEIGHT LOSS AND IMPROVING OVERALL HEALTH.

CHRISTINE PINE

CONTENTS

The groundwork of all happiness is health.

— LEIGH HUNT

INTRODUCTION

How many different kinds of diets have you tried in the past? More than one, right? The one thing they all seem to have in common is temporary results. I don't know about you, but I always struggled to maintain my weight-loss results with different diets. They either didn't fit with my lifestyle, or they were expensive to do. The one main downside to all the diets I have tried is as soon as you stop them, the weight piles back on. We all have busy lives looking after our families and balancing our careers. Adding a diet plan to all of this requires calorie counting, expensive supplements, and weekly weigh-ins. It's just too much added pressure. We spend weeks balancing everything in our lives, and in the end, it can become too much. Even if you aren't on a diet, it can become soul-crushing when we try to eat well, but there just doesn't seem time to balance our lives with healthy eating.

The weekends aren't much better. Exhausted from the insanity of the week, all you want to do is relax in front of the television and binge-watch your favorite shows. You grab whatever is available in the pantry to eat, then you settle in to enjoy. Before you know it, a new week has started, and you have done little to change your diet and activity levels.

This may seem like a problem only you are facing, but it's a global epidemic. Low activity, coupled with foods high in processed fats and refined sugars are creating a generation of overweight and more worryingly, obese individuals. This is by no means a statistic to fat-shame or scare anyone. Life is hectic enough without having the added worry about getting a balanced diet and exercise; however, it isn't something you should be ignoring.

A healthy body is a balance between our diet and how much we exercise. While most doctors tend to prescribe 150 minutes of moderate exercise with two days of strength training, this isn't always possible. Where are you supposed to find all this time to hit the gym? A fast-paced life can make up for a lack of dedicated exercise time, but more often than not, unfortunately it doesn't.

As for food, you should be eating a diet containing all the nutrients, vitamins, minerals, carbohydrates, fats, and proteins to fuel your body. However, a perfect body isn't just about what exercise you do and the food you eat, it's about adopting a lifestyle that can help achieve it.

HEALTHY LIFESTYLE

A healthy lifestyle is one where everything you do benefits your body. Remember, what you do to your body at a young age will affect it later in your life. This is why it's vital to keep an eye on what you eat and your activity levels, but these aren't the only parts of your life you should be monitoring.

Sleeping well is very important and should be at the top of your list to achieve a good body condition. Your body needs sleep, as, without rest, your body cannot repair day-to-day damage. Poor quality sleep makes you feel tired and unable to do anything—especially after a tough day. A good night's rest depends on being active and eating well.

Feeling good about yourself is something many people take for granted. When you're happy about yourself, your mental health improves. This will do wonders for your confidence and self-esteem. However, when you aren't happy with yourself, your mindfulness suffers.

When you are mindful of things in your life, it's easier to deal with daily stress. Stress is everywhere, you can't avoid it, so you must manage it. However, with poor sleep, diet, and no activity, this task becomes a mountain most people can't summit. The strain on your body could lead to heart disease, organ issues (such as stomach ulcers), high blood pressure, and lead you to make poor decisions—usually with choices about your diet. Most people won't reach for a healthy snack when they feel down, they reach for the closest sugary treat and avoid going to the gym.

A healthy lifestyle is about bringing everything into balance: diet, exercise, mindfulness, and good quality sleep. By doing this, you get many benefits. This includes better health, longevity (longer life), increased confidence, higher self-esteem, and help to combat stress. These are hardly your only benefits. With a healthy body, you can combat infertility (high cholesterol can lower it), protect your eyesight (high blood pressure damages your eyes), and help you to avoid daily addictions as you manage negative outlets and choices when you're feeling bad.

HEALTHY WEIGHT

Many people assume a healthy weight means they are healthy, and technically they aren't wrong. Yet, many women go about getting to their ideal weight the wrong way. Every year there is a new fad diet with many celebrities who praise it. Then, millions of women try these diets with little to no results for the majority of them. In some cases, these fad diets can cause an increase in weight, increasing the already growing population of obese women.

Obesity is a global trend that's increasing certain cancers, heart disease, type 2 diabetes, and many other conditions. Yet, how can you lose weight safely without it coming back to haunt you? This is a difficult question to answer, and many women give up. Getting to the ideal weight is difficult, as it requires commitment. Losing it too quickly is also bad for you. It's recommended that you lose no more than 1–2 pounds a week, as this is more sustainable in the long run.

When overweight, losing as little as 5% of your weight will show a marked improvement in your health. It'll increase your energy levels, make you more mobile, and increase your mood and self-confidence. What lady doesn't love someone noticing that she's lost a few pounds?

You may be thinking that's easier said than done, but it's not. To lose the weight and keep it off, you need to change the current lifestyle you are living. The best way I have found to lose weight is through intermittent fasting.

MY STORY

Like so many of us, I have a busy lifestyle that leaves little time to concentrate on what really matters... my health. Over the last few years, I have tried many different diets, juices, potions and plans, but nothing ever worked for me or became a lifestyle that I could stick with, long term.

Whatever I tried worked for a while, but it was always a struggle to keep up with the diets and being forced to cut out the foods I loved was just too hard. Yes, I saw results in weight loss, but the one common issue I faced was when the diet stopped, the weight piled back on. This became an endless cycle of diet, struggle, deprivation, hunger, sadness and the inevitable failure. What was the point in battling to lose the weight, whilst cutting out the foods I enjoyed, only to see little results that would be reversed as soon as I stopped the dieting? Each new diet was another piece of my willower and happiness chipped away until finally reaching the point where I just didn't want to try any more.

Standing 5'4" and weighing 175 pounds, I stumbled across Intermittent Fasting. To start with I suffered from the same doubts as with all the other diets I had tried, and thought to myself, how could this be any different than all the rest? I decided to give dieting one more try and researched this technique.

The science behind the technique gave me hope and this really did look like a lifestyle that I could convert to, whilst balancing my busy schedule, and I am so glad I did. Never really having time for breakfast, or enjoying it, I decided to try the 16:8 plan. I stopped eating breakfast and had my first meal at 12pm each day. To be honest, my breakfasts before this consisted of a quick fruit juice and maybe some cereal or toast, if I had time. Knowing what I know now, this is the worst way I could have started my day and it's even more frustrating that I didn't even want breakfast, I just had it as that's what we do, right? We eat as soon as we can in the morning.

I changed my breakfast to a black cup of coffee, as once I had researched fasting, I knew this would not break my fast, and it would give me a quick pick-me-up first thing. Then around 12pm I would have a light lunch, normally a salad or a sandwich with a low-calorie soda. Then in the evening, around 6pm I would have my main meal. I started by eating what I knew, as that was easy for me, but over time I introduced more healthy unprocessed foods.

I was still snacking, but I would always stop eating before 8pm, which gave me the perfect 16:8 window. To be honest, I didn't really struggle at all with this way of eating and over time I started introducing more healthy snacks, such as nuts and fruits that were lower in sugar, such as strawberries and blueberries. The one thing that I couldn't quite get my head around was the fact that I wasn't depriving myself and therefore was not experiencing the same battles I faced with all the other diets I had tried and failed over the years.

I started intermittent fasting back in 2019 and I am still going strong. This is now my lifestyle and I have no intentions of stopping and to be honest… I don't want to. The weight keeps coming off, month after month and I have now lost over 40 pounds and the most important thing is, I feel so much better physically, but most importantly, mentally. I have noticed such a change in my body shape and the fat has reduced significantly. The clothes in my wardrobe, that had been relegated to the darkest corners now fit me and I no longer have to keep the larger sizes, for when the weight gain comes back. Because it doesn't come back!

Occasionally I stop eating at 6pm, which extends my eating window to 18:6, but I don't do this every day.

Also, there are times where I might need to eat past 8pm, maybe at the weekend, if I am going out with friends, but I don't worry. The next day I am back on track and this works for me. I don't do this often but it gives me the freedom to live my life, whilst still following the intermittent fasting lifestyle.

I wish I could talk to each and every one of you about just how great intermittent fasting is, and what it has done for me. I hope my book gives you the inspiration and information you need to start your new lifestyle and like me, never look back!

WHY INTERMITTENT FASTING

Intermittent fasting wasn't like other diets I had tried in the past. It didn't require calorie counting or restricting what I could eat. I didn't need to buy special food, and I could do all of it from the comfort of my home.

Many studies show that intermittent fasting aids in lowering the risk of many diseases, helps to maintain a healthy weight, and therefore allows for better mental health. I figured why not try it and see what happens. All I had to lose was the weight, after all.

After following intermittent fasting for over 2 years, I lost and kept off 40 pounds. I now look and feel better than I have in years. My fat content is down, I can move as I want, and now have the body shape I am happy with.

The best thing about intermittent fasting? There are several techniques you can use. If you find one to be too difficult, choose another. The most important aspect is focusing on when you can and can't eat, not what you may or may not eat! Anyone can try this lifestyle change without spending a fortune.

WHO SHOULD AVOID FASTING

Intermittent fasting is a lifestyle change that is easy to follow, but it's not for everyone. Some individuals should give this a skip for their health:

- Anyone under the age of 18.
- Pregnant or breastfeeding mothers, as this could affect the baby or the quality of milk produced.
- People who suffer from type 1 diabetes.
- Those with an eating disorder.
- People who have to take medication after eating.
- Those who are underweight, frail, or elderly.

If you're still unsure, consult your doctor. Fasting isn't a diet, it's a lifestyle change—one you can start today! So why wait? Turn the page to educate yourself about how one change can improve many aspects of your life!

Nothing is impossible. The word itself says 'I'm possible!'

— AUDREY HEPBURN

1

DEFINING INTERMITTENT FASTING

Y ou have likely heard about intermittent fasting before and have thought it nothing more than a fad diet. However, it isn't a fad diet, it's just a change in your lifestyle, and it has already helped many people in the past. So, what makes intermittent fasting popular? Let's learn all about it.

WHAT IS INTERMITTENT FASTING?

While most diets govern what and how much you are allowed to eat, intermittent fasting only limits when you may eat. When you are allowed to eat will depend on which of the fasting techniques you want to try. This lifestyle is nothing new to the human race. Before we had refrigerators, before we even had farms, ancient humans were hunter-gatherers. These nomadic people would move from one place to another, keeping on the heels of the migratory animals they hunted. Hunting requires a large investment of energy, and humans weren't always successful. This is why those that didn't join the hunt, gathered what edibles they could while they traveled. These foods could be anything from fruits and vegetables to roots and nuts. However, there was no guarantee that these foods would be available in the areas the humans were traveling through. If the hunters missed a catch and the gatherers couldn't find anything to eat, the tribe was likely to go hungry that night.

Yet, the human species is still around, and they didn't starve to death. We are built to skip meals now and again when there isn't enough food around. However, with the discovery of agriculture—some 12,000 years ago—we have become spoiled for food as it's now more readily available to us. Now with fridges, freezers, and shopping centers, we rarely go hungry as we are surrounded by food all the time. Because of this, humans have started eating more and become less active.

Intermittent fasting—also known as IF—is when a person sets cycles of eating and fasting. Some fasting times are more extreme than others, but the general rule is that the longer you don't eat, the more weight you can potentially lose. All within reason, of course. Fasting isn't always about losing weight; some use it for detox, spiritual, or religious reasons. Religions such as Islam, Buddhism, and Christianity believe that with the help of fasting, people can cleanse their souls.

HISTORY OF INTERMITTENT FASTING

Many ancient Greeks believed that when they ate food, there was a chance they would also welcome a demon into their bodies, which needed to be purged in some manner. This manner was by fasting.

The ancient Greeks believed that fasting was the body's way of dealing with many diseases while increasing cognitive abilities. Think about the last time you ate until you had a full belly. Did you suddenly have the energy to deal with the day? Likely not. Full bellies tend to make people sleepy. This is why there are so many Sunday lunchtime naps! Fasting was seen as an ancient healing technique, supported by many famous Greeks such as Aristotle, Pythagoras, and Plato. Aside from healing, fasting was also used to bring about visions and powerful dreams.

Fasting as a means to remain healthy was steadfastly believed all around the world for thousands of years.

This wasn't something that was taught around the world, but rather developed naturally as humans experienced the world around them. Each culture would have unique ways of explaining why they did it—communing with gods or having visions—or how it came about.

However, as humans started to develop, an interesting theory about disease came to light. In the mid-1800s, it was believed that many diseases were caused by an excess of eating, which led to increased gastric juices. Many scientific observations from this time to the late 1950s noted that when overweight or obese people started fasting, they lost weight, and their lives improved. Doctors began prescribing fasting as a tool to help these types of people lose weight and live healthier lifestyles.

One such success story occurred in 1965. Angus Barbieri was a 27-year-old man who weighed 456 pounds. Angus, realizing his weight would kill him sooner than later, decided to set himself a weight goal of 180 pounds. Under the daily supervision of doctors and a strict diet of non-nutritional drinks (zero-calorie) and vitamins, he now holds the world record for the most weight lost while fasting. He lost an astounding 276 pounds in 382 days.

However, fasting to this extreme level should be discussed with a doctor and closely monitored.

Fasting studies continued with human volunteers throughout the 1950s and have made a comeback in the last few years. This is because while human studies are few and far between, the studies on laboratory rodents have continued since the 1940s. It is through these studies that we see many benefits occurring in the lab models. However, we cannot draw direct comparisons between what we see in mice and what could happen in humans. More human studies should be conducted by scientists to prove the benefits of intermittent fasting.

SCIENCE BEHIND INTERMITTENT FASTING

Although many fasting benefits are anecdotal, science can explain why it does work, and it's surprisingly straightforward. The idea behind intermittent fasting is to "starve" your body for a set time. Most people eat 2,000–2,500 calories every day, usually as three meals and two snacks. During intermittent fasting, there isn't enough time to eat all these calories, so you are forced to eat less food. Less food means you have access to less energy coming into your body. When the body doesn't get this energy supply, it has to resort to an internal one.

When you eat food that contains carbohydrates, these are broken down to glucose. Glucose is then absorbed into the bloodstream and sent to the various organs and muscles that require it to function. When eating a balanced diet, there is rarely an excess of glucose. However, when in excess, it's then stored as glycogen and fat in the liver and adipose (fat) tissue. However, fat is required by the body to function normally, so having some in your body is necessary.

Once you are no longer eating, the liver breaks down its glycogen and then releases the glucose back into the bloodstream. It can take roughly 10–12 hours for an inactive person to burn through the liver's stored glycogen. An active person will do this much quicker. If the body still requires more energy, the adipose tissue is targeted next. The fat is broken down into fatty acids that go to the liver to make ketones. Ketones are the alternative energy source to glucose, and your body can readily run on them—as seen with the keto diet. Your body will continue to use up the excess fat until you feed it once more and give it more glucose.

When fasting is done correctly, you will lose weight, drop high blood pressure, lower your cholesterol, increase your brain's health, and fight back against the onset of type 2 diabetes.

The hormone insulin is in charge of getting cells to accept glucose. As soon as glucose is absorbed into your bloodstream, expect insulin to be released soon after. However, when you eat too often or too much, there is too much glucose for insulin to manage. This leads the pancreas to secrete more and more insulin to get the job done. Over time, if you have too much insulin, the cells become resistant or desensitized to it, resulting in insulin not working the way it should. This is known as insulin insensitivity—also known as insulin resistance. When you are suffering from this, it's the start of prediabetes, which can become type 2 diabetes if ignored long enough. With fasting, you are lowering how often you're introducing glucose into your blood and lowering the insulin response to it, helping you fight against diabetes.

Even your brain gets a boost when you are fasting. During the fasting process, there is an increase in brain-derived neurotrophic factors (BDNF). This protein is vital in the growth of new nervous tissue, aiding in the growth and longevity of neurons.

There is also a change in the hormones you produce. Human growth hormones (HGH) and norepinephrine (fat-burning hormone) increase the longer you fast. As norepinephrine increases, so does your metabolic rate, which in turn aids in weight loss. Meanwhile, HGH helps to maintain your muscles during fasting and increases cellular repair and metabolism.

With all these benefits, you are likely left with the question of how long should you fast? While fasting for extended periods can be harmful, the more frequently you fast for shorter times, the easier it becomes. No one way of fasting is perfect for everyone, and some techniques are better suited for men than women. Being without food for hours may seem daunting at first, but if you place the majority of your fasting time during your sleep, it'll be much easier. When you start, you may also find you are low on energy, so reduce the amount of fitness training you may be doing. The effects of prolonged fasting are discussed further in Chapter 2.

EFFECTIVENESS

Intermittent fasting is only as effective as your willpower to stick to the technique you want to try. In most human studies, many people would drop out because they couldn't adhere to the fasting technique outlined in the study.

In most cases, while intermittent fasting, you can drop your energy intake from 60–100%. Most women get no benefit from cutting their energy intake by 100% when trying the alternate-day fasting technique. However, that is not to say this will affect all women the same. It's best to choose a technique that suits you and the lifestyle you lead. Once you're comfortable with the technique you're trying, it'll be much easier to continue it for longer.

As for the results, it depends on how you prefer to fast, what you eat during the eating period, and whether you decide to exercise or not. The main thing to remember is that your body will give you signs when it can't take anymore. Listen to it closely. It will tell you if you are fasting too long or if you need a specific type of meal to fuel you.

Review your diet. Although you don't need to drastically cut foods out, you should concentrate on putting better fuel into your body. In Chapter 10, there are many recipes for you to try to aid your fasting quest. If you find letting go of unhealthy food is hard, you need to ask yourself why this is. Many women tend to overeat because of their emotional attachment to food. This attachment can be tough to break, and you may need some help. Food addiction is as bad as obesity, but luckily there are some professionals (home doctors or psychologists) who can help you.

Science is still divided on the effectiveness of fasting, but anecdotal evidence from many people fasting shows that it is effective for them. At the end of the day, you won't know if it's effective if you don't give it a try.

SUCCESS STORIES

Still don't believe that intermittent fasting is good for you? Here are a few success stories:

Miroch52 (2017) states that they tried the 16:8 fasting technique, and now it has become a complete lifestyle change for them. They do occasionally get hungry 30 minutes after waking. However, they ignore the feeling and go about preparing for their day, forgetting about being hungry until lunchtime. They say this technique helped them overcome eating when bored.

Another user of Reddit, who goes by the name of chips15, mentions that they would wake up every morning to have cheese and an egg on toast before starting their day (chips15, 2017). However, after switching to intermittent fasting, they found that they no longer needed to have breakfast, preferring to only eat again in the afternoon.

AshKals practices a different kind of fasting technique. They only eat from 8 a.m. to 3 p.m., then fast through supper until the following morning (AshKals, 2017). They found that this prevented them from binge eating when they started to relax. They manage to control their hunger by having well-balanced breakfasts and large lunches. When they know that they will have to have dinner, they simply skip breakfast and only eat again the next afternoon.

STARTING INTERMITTENT FASTING: WHERE TO BEGIN?

The most challenging part of any lifestyle change is where to start. You may already have reviewed your food at home and decided to cut most of it from your diet. Stop! Remember that intermittent fasting isn't just about what you eat but about when you eat. That occasional slice of cake? You may have it, as long as it's occasionally. Food viewed as junk food is still fuel for your body, although not necessarily the best type.

A diet for fasting needs to include food that is nutrient-dense, high in fiber, contains good fats, and has lean protein. Now that it'll be more difficult to have a large quantity of food every day, you need to consider the quality of what you eat. You're not only fueling your body, but you're also providing sustenance for your gut microbes. Keeping them happy will ensure your body remains healthy during your fasting periods.

So, what can you eat and drink during your eating periods? You're spoiled for choice. Here are some examples to help you make the right choices:

Fats

- Unsaturated fats are the best fats you can have in your diet. While you may want to reach for some olive or canola oil, also consider adding avocado to your diet. This fruit is high in unsaturated fats, minerals, vitamins, and fiber. It is guaranteed to make you feel fuller for longer.
- Nuts also contain unsaturated fats and fiber. They make wonderful snacks or additions to salads.
- Regardless of the health benefits of unsaturated fats, ensure that you don't have too much in your diet as they are high in calories.

Protein

- Eggs are fantastic as they can be prepared in many different ways. They are high in protein, good cholesterol, and easy to prepare.
- Lean poultry and fish should make up more of your diet than red meat. The combination of

omega-fatty acids is perfect for making you feel full long after you have eaten.

- Fish and seafood are high in vitamin D, which is needed to make strong muscles, bones, and teeth.
- Consider having a meatless dish now and again with tofu or tempeh.
- Don't forget your legumes such as beans, peas, and chickpeas. Legumes are a great source of protein and fiber while remaining low in carbohydrates.

Vegetables

- The darker green a vegetable is, the better it is for you.
- Brassica or cruciferous vegetables such as cauliflower, broccoli, Brussels sprouts, and cabbage are high in fiber. Not only do they make your stomach feel fuller, but they ensure you remain regular.
- Generally, you want to avoid starchy vegetables, but don't discredit potatoes—especially jacketed potatoes. They are high in fiber, vitamins, and minerals, as long as you don't enjoy them as French fries, chips, or smothered in butter or sour cream.

Fruit

- All fruit contains sugar; there is no way to avoid it, so manage your portions.
- Berries are generally lower in sugar and go great with Greek yogurt as a snack.
- Fruits are full of flavonoids which have many health benefits and antioxidant effects.

Grains

- It's best to avoid processed grains such as white bread or rice.
- Whole grains give you more fiber than processed varieties.
- Grains as a whole will have a lot of carbohydrates. However, with the higher fiber content, glucose is released slower, preventing a sudden glucose spike.
- Don't stick to what you know! Try grains such as bulgur, millet, and sorghum to challenge your tastebuds!

Dairy

- Enjoy as long as it is low-fat, or eat full-fat in moderation.

- Yogurt should be enjoyed unsweetened where possible.

Beverages

- When fasting, stick to fresh water. This can seem a little boring at first, but luckily there are some things you can add to make it more exciting.
- Add a twist of lemon, some fresh mint leaves, and maybe a slice or two of cucumber to encourage you to drink more water. If this isn't exciting enough, try unsweetened, unflavored soda water.
- Some people can't function without a cup of coffee or tea in the morning. You can still enjoy your morning beverage, as long as during your fast, you aren't adding sugar, sweetener, milk, or cream to your drink.

Occasionally, a change in diet can cause stomach issues. Add probiotics, such as yogurt, kombucha, or sauerkraut, to your diet to bolster the microbes in your intestines.

Play around with different foods to see which allow you to make it through your fasting period without hunger pangs. What suits me, may not suit you. Experiment until you find the perfect fit for the fasting technique you plan on using.

Then we come to the part I know everyone is dreading. What about our favorite junk food? Everything eaten should be in moderation, but realize that most junk foods aren't nutrient-dense or have the fiber to sustain you through a fasting period. Try to avoid the following foods and drinks.

- Baked goods, jams and jellies, and candies as they are high in refined sugar.
- Fruit juice is highly-processed fruit that is literally pure sugar water with no fiber.
- Any sweetened drinks, as these are generally sweetened with corn syrup.
- All sugary cereals
- All trans fats

Learn to read the back of the nutritional labels to see what you are really putting into your body when you eat something. In the following chapter, we'll look more in-depth at what happens the longer you fast, how women are affected by fasting, and possible side effects you could experience.

Do not allow people to dim your shine because they are blinded. Tell them to put some sunglasses on.

— LADY GAGA

2

WHAT FASTING DOES TO YOU

F asting is more than not eating. It's about the changes you'll get to experience.

WHAT HAPPENS WHEN YOU FAST

Have you ever considered what would happen if you missed more than a meal? Sure, you'd feel hungry, but what happens inside your body? The more time you spend fasting, the more changes your body will undergo.

After Eight Hours

Most people can easily achieve eight hours of fasting, as they generally sleep through it. As you sleep, no new glucose is being consumed, so there is no need for insulin to spike. Your body turns to glycogen mostly and some fat to keep it functioning. As you start to wake, you immediately think you need something to eat, even if you aren't hungry. That's because we've been indoctrinated to believe we can only get through the day if we eat breakfast. However, you should never force yourself to eat if you aren't hungry. If you aren't hungry at this stage, give breakfast a skip and see how long you can last before you start feeling hunger gnawing at you.

After 12 Hours

Only four hours later, your body continues to use glycogen and fat to fuel itself. Glycogen is starting to run out at this stage, and your body is ramping up the fat burning. You may or may not begin to feel hungry now. It'll depend on how large your previous meal was the night before and what it consisted of.

There is an increase in human growth hormone (HGH), which helps increase the metabolism, but that isn't the only thing it does. This hormone gives an anti-aging effect and aids in fat burning. It's also in charge of making new proteins and healing any damage to joints.

After 18 Hours

Glucose levels in the blood are starting to run low with no new carbohydrates to replace them. Certain body parts require glucose to function correctly, so the body needs to find it somewhere. Through gluconeogenesis, the liver uses non-carbohydrates—such as lactate or amino acids—to make glucose. Your body is moving away from glycogen—hoping to store some for an emergency—and relying on fat as its main energy source.

To save on resources, your body goes through what is known as autophagy—which is also known as self-eating. As horrific as this sounds, it's completely normal and has many benefits. Through autophagy, your body uses old and damaged proteins and any harmful viruses and bacteria it finds. By doing this, the body uses waste products and reduces the number of potentially harmful microbes. Because of autophagy, the immune system becomes boosted, and the brain suffers from less inflammation. Without periods of fasting the body rarely has a chance to self-clean as it's constantly being fed.

There is a decrease in advanced glycation end products (AGEs) which are known to damage proteins, therefore aiding in healing. This helps to prevent the creation of amyloid plaques—a collection of misfolded proteins—from occurring in the brain. These plaques are one of the factors behind Alzheimer's and other neurodegenerative diseases.

As your body uses more fat, more ketones are being produced. These are an alternative source of energy that the body can thrive on. Ketones are less inflammatory than glucose—especially when following a low-carbohydrate diet. This energy source can also be used by the brain, as this organ can function on ketones and glucose.

There is an increase in brain-derived neurotrophic factor (BDNF) and HGH. The BDNF—as it helps to create new connections in the brain—will help you to focus and learn easier. The HGH at this stage helps regulate the fat metabolism, but after a few more hours, its function changes.

You may start noticing you are hungry at this stage. Some people who are used to fasting for long periods can shrug it off, while others may drink some water to help them get past the worst of the hunger pangs. Feeling hungry is normal. If you feel you have fasted enough, you can gently break your fast with a small meal, or maybe a snack, before a larger meal several hours later. If you feel confident enough to extend your fast, then do so.

After 24 Hours

After a day of not eating, autophagy increases as your body tries to recycle as much as possible to prevent energy loss. The body is no longer using glycogen as an energy source but instead only using fat and making glucose through gluconeogenesis. If you are suffering from a fatty liver, your body will use this fat to refuel it. Ketones in the blood are now at a nutritional level, enough to maintain your body's energy needs and helps to suppress appetite.

Gluconeogenesis is now targeting the glycerol backbone in the triglycerides (a type of fat) as a way to make glucose. What remains of the triglyceride is the fatty acids, which are used to make more ketones. Your body is also looking to replenish its protein stores, so it recycles waste proteins and any free-floating protein. Thanks to the HGH, your muscles are not being broken down to make protein or glucose.

The hunger is more noticeable now. You will need to ask yourself if this is just a feeling because of a routine you are used to, or if you can't go on with your fasting. Hunger comes and goes and can be managed by drinking water. This is the stage you can start to train yourself to do longer fasting periods if you want to. Some doctors believe that an extended fasting period is good for your body now and again. If you can push yourself a little longer, do so, but there is no need to.

High levels of insulin can cause inflammation throughout the body. Now that there is less inflammation, your body has time to heal from the constant strain. Even your gut (stomach and intestines) has an opportunity to heal. With no meals constantly needing to be digested, the organs aren't working as hard and can get a well-deserved rest.

When it comes to exercise, it's best to give high-intensity workouts a skip on days you plan to go without food for 24 hours. You can still take a gentle walk if you feel up to it.

After 48 Hours

When planning a fasting session lasting longer than 24 hours, you'll need to remain hydrated and consider supplementing minerals (sodium and potassium) and a vitamin B complex. Minerals are constantly being used and flushed from your body and will need to be replaced. Many vitamins are needed to run the body efficiently, and when not present, you can suffer side effects.

The hunger is now nagging at you constantly, but luckily the worst is only during the first half of the second day. If you can manage to keep it at bay long enough, it'll disappear after some time, making the rest of your day easier to overcome.

At this stage of fasting, the HGH and BDFN are operating at almost 500% of their base level (Dr. Sten

Ekberg, 2022). Ketones are now at a therapeutic level. Your body's autophagy is close to running optimally, as it continues to look for resources to recycle to fuel your energy levels. For people who suffer from insulin resistance, this is when you start making the cells sensitive to insulin once more. There should be little to no insulin present in your blood. Your body is now receiving most of its energy requirements from fat and some from glycerol.

Up to this point, you may find you can exercise with no problem. However, now it is becoming too difficult to do high-intensity training. Anaerobic exercises—such as running, swimming, and extended High-Intensity Interval Training (HIIT)—require oxygen and a lot of glucose to fuel the muscles and organs as you train. After 48 hours, there isn't any more glucose except for the glycogen in the liver. However, this is meant for emergencies when a boost of energy is needed. If you push yourself, you may find that you are too exhausted, and your body will turn to your muscles to produce glucose. If you want to exercise, it's best to take walks that don't elevate your heart rate too much.

After 72 Hours

Fasting for this long isn't the norm, and should only be done a few times a year and after some fasting practice.

You will need additional minerals to keep your body functioning the way it should.

At this stage, your body will experience better levels of autophagy. With all the work done to clear up waste products in the body; this is when the body starts to reverse some of the damage that has occurred due to poor lifestyle choices. This includes type 2 diabetes, cardiovascular disease, and high blood pressure, and offers some protection from certain cancers.

Your body will also experience hematopoietic stem cell regeneration. These are specific stem cells that can become any type of blood cell. With this regeneration of these stem cells, you can see an increase in newly made white blood cells. This leads to boosting your immune system.

After 72 hours of not eating, it starts getting difficult to ignore the hunger pains. You may also find that you're struggling to concentrate, have headaches, and feel exhausted. The moment you start feeling poorly, it's time to break your fast with a small, nutrient-dense meal. You should never push yourself to the point of feeling ill. Fasting is about gradually reaching the duration of not eating, not to stop eating completely.

As exercise stresses the heart, lungs, and muscles to make them stronger, so does fasting for your cells.

They will first be stressed at not getting their usual energy supply, but in time, they will get used to it. They will adapt and become strong enough for you to fast as long as you see fit. It's best to stick to shorter fasting times as a lifestyle change rather than attempting multi-day fasting periods.

MEN VERSUS WOMEN

Men and women differ in looks, hormones produced, and even have different nutritional needs. Because of this, their bodies will react differently when going through a fasting period. There are no human studies as of yet that compare obese men and women against each other to see how they react to different fasting techniques. Of the human fasting studies done, the only fasting techniques that have been explored are alternate-day fasting and time-restricted eating (16:8).

One study we can use for comparison was done in 2012 and used non-obese men and women for three weeks on an alternating fasting period. At the end of 22 days, it was found that men had an improvement in their insulin sensitivity, while women had a decrease.

Other human studies have shown that men tend to get a boosted metabolism within 24 hours, while women don't get the same boost. Generally, in women, the metabolism slows, and it's believed that this may be a way to conserve energy and store fat as the body is convinced there is a famine. Women also tended to be hungrier after 24 hours and in some occurrences, it was found that extended fasting contributed to obesity and diabetes.

Even the mice models in the study by Freire et al. (2020) showed that the female mice performed worse on a 12-week alternate-day fasting program than the males. Although they did lose 19% of their starting weight, they had smaller ovaries and larger adrenal glands. All of which point to chronic stress and hormonal dysfunction.

However, before getting discouraged by science, you should be asking yourself, why? Why aren't women getting the same results as men? It comes down to our hormones and possibly the structure of female livers.

Some studies have suggested that how livers regulate glucose may be different between the two genders as they fast. Female pancreases also tend to release less glucagon in response to exercise when glucose is needed to fuel the body. It would seem that women struggle to clear glucose as efficiently as men while fasting. This may be because of how we metabolize carbohydrates. This isn't only driven by our lifestyle and body compositions but also by the sex hormones produced. Women produce more kisspeptin—which is in charge of puberty, controlling fertility, and regulating the sex hormones. It also makes a person sensitive to changes in their energy balance. Once our energy levels dip below a certain point, kisspeptin causes women to react quicker to hunger than men. Meaning the more your energy dips, the hungrier you'll feel, and you may want to reach for a snack. This is why women should be careful when fasting for more than 24 hours at a stretch. It's possible, but it'll take some planning to achieve.

HOW TO FAST AS A WOMAN

Women can certainly get the benefits of fasting, but they may not be able to achieve the same results as men —especially with the longer fasting times. Upon choosing your preferred fasting technique—see Chapter 4—don't just jump in and assume you'll manage it. Fasting requires some practice, and it's wise to try for a few days out of the week before making the lifestyle switch totally.

When a technique doesn't work for you—for whatever reason—pick a new one. It needs to suit your needs, and you shouldn't force yourself. As a woman, your menstrual cycle will affect how you feel when fasting, as you may need a few extra calories to get through it.

You may want to change your fasting time to help you or change your diet a little to get as much protein and iron as possible.

Not all lifestyle changes are positive, and there is a chance that fasting for too long can have a negative effect on your cycle. Extensive or extreme fasting has been known to cause anxiety, irregular or missed periods resulting in lowering the chance of pregnancy, and sleep disturbances. If you experience any of these side effects, you should review how you fast and your diet to compensate.

CELEBRITY SUCCESSES

To help you overcome your nervousness about the side effects of fasting, here are some success stories about celebrities who have tried intermittent fasting, and how it worked for them.

Chris Pratt, who on his Twitter account in 2018, told his fans about his journey with intermittent fasting. With all the action movies he does, he is required to stay in shape. How he achieved this was usually through a strict diet and exercise. He decided to try intermittent fasting by skipping breakfast and only eating again at lunchtime. With intermittent fasting, he even gets to enjoy a cup of black coffee in the morning.

After trying the diet, he managed to lose weight and still managed to do his cardio training in the morning.

Despite this diet change not being as strict as others he had followed in the past, he's still careful about what he eats after a fast. He believes that following a well-balanced diet instead of gorging after a fast is a healthy way of approaching the end of the non-eating period.

He isn't the only celebrity to swear by intermittent fasting. Jack Dorsey limits himself to a single meal a day, high in protein and vegetables, to see him through to the following day. He's even able to do some light exercise eating this way.

The women of Hollywood also love intermittent fasting. Jennifer Aniston uses the 16:8 fasting technique six days a week while reserving her Sunday as a day she can be more lenient. Eating this way powers her five-times-a-week training schedule with no problem. Molly Sims is an advocate for a 12-hour fasting period. She believes that fasting is a way to reset one's metabolism.

STARTING INTERMITTENT: UNDERSTANDING WEIGHT CONTROL HORMONES

Weight control is a little more complex than what, when, and how much you eat. It boils down to the hormones the body produces. Hormones are secreted by the endocrine system through many organs throughout your body. Depending on which one is secreted, it has a specific function. Many hormones can help fight or encourage obesity if they are in excess or deficient:

Adiponectin

- This hormone is found in fat tissue.
- It helps to boost metabolism without increasing the feeling of hunger.

Cholecystokinin (CCK)

- This hormone is secreted by the gut when the stomach is full.
- It increases the release of leptin and aids in making proteins and boosting digestion.

Cortisol

- Cortisol is considered the stress hormone and is secreted by the adrenal glands.
- It controls the fat and carbohydrate metabolism.
- Cortisol is responsible for the quick release of energy when a fight or flight situation is

encountered. However, afterward, a person experiences an increase in appetite and cravings leading to overeating.

- Cortisol production is triggered by anything that causes stress, such as exercise or a lack of sleep.

Sex hormones

- Women secrete estrogen from ovaries, while men secrete androgens from testes.
- These hormones determine where the fat is distributed in the body. More fat around your middle increases the risk of stroke and heart disease.
- As people age, their sex hormone production changes, changing the fat distribution.
- The lower the hormone, the higher the chance of weight increase.

Ghrelin

- When the stomach is empty, it secretes this hormone to stimulate appetite. It also influences your sleep patterns.
- The higher the concentration of this hormone, the hungrier you will feel.

Glucagon-like peptide-1 (GLP-1)

- The small intestine is responsible for the secretion of this hormone.
- It keeps blood sugar stable and promotes the feeling of fullness.

HGH

- This hormone comes from the pituitary gland and increases metabolism.

Insulin

- The pancreas secretes this hormone, which causes cells to accept glucose.

Leptin

- The white adipose tissue secretes this hormone.
- It helps to increase metabolism and fat storage while reducing appetite.

Neuropeptide Y (NPY)

- This hormone is mostly created and released by neurons.

- It helps to stimulate appetite and lower energy usage while fasting or in times of stress.

Peptide YY (PYY)

- Similar to GLP-1, this hormone is secreted by the small intestine.
- It helps to lower appetite.

Low activity and poor diet can cause the body to reset how its hormones function. Instead of suppressing hunger and distributing fat correctly, these hormones may increase weight, leading to obesity and other diseases. When a person is obese, hormones such as estrogen or androgens, GLP-1, and PYY are lower than they should be. However, when hormones such as leptin, insulin, NPY, and CCK are high, the body's cells become resistant to reacting to them. This phenomenon is seen in many people who suffer from obesity.

I'm not going to continue knocking that old door that doesn't open for me. I'm going to create my own door and walk through that.

— AVA DUVERNAY

3

FALLACIES AND FACTS OF FASTING

There are many fallacies when it comes to intermittent fasting and a healthy diet. Have you been told that you can eat whatever you want if you're fasting and you will definitely lose weight? Or maybe you've heard that your metabolism will slow down if you fast. How about the old classic; if you don't eat breakfast your day will be a disaster?

These are just some examples of misinformation that have been spread to scare you off from trying any fasting technique to lose weight. Fasting is an exercise in getting your body into a calorie deficit and is dependent on the kind of food you eat while fasting, although occasional naughty foods are okay. You can't expect your body to burn through calories when you're downing sodas, pizzas, and burgers before and after your fast, on a regular basis. Intermittent fasting goes hand in hand with a healthy diet to be effective. Let's delve a little deeper into some facts and fiction about fasting.

MYTHS

There are many myths surrounding fasting which are not only false but can be detrimental to your health if you keep believing in them. Let's start with the beliefs surrounding eating frequent meals.

It's believed that eating frequent meals will boost your metabolism, help you to not feel hungry, and lose weight. These are all myths. Consuming frequent meals increases the chance of overeating and keeping insulin constantly in the bloodstream. This doesn't increase the metabolism. It doesn't lower cravings or feelings of hunger. Small frequent meals may contribute to increased feelings of hunger over time, as you are training your body to expect meals more often. Lastly, there is no evidence that frequent meals will help you lose weight.

What about breakfast? For decades we have heard that breakfast is the most important meal of the day, and skipping it can lead to increased weight, hunger, and cravings. Also, not true. Unless the breakfast is well-balanced with the necessary nutrients to do a specific task, it isn't needed. Most people aren't even hungry when they wake up!

The brain needing glucose to function optimally is another old myth. The brain indeed needs glucose to function but it doesn't need you feeding it glucose to do so. The brain can function well on ketones and glucose can be made through gluconeogenesis.

Even protein consumption has a myth. It's believed that a person can only digest 30 grams of protein in one sitting, regardless of how much they eat. This is why a protein meal needs to be eaten every 2–3 hours. Completely untrue. Your body will digest and use what protein you give it during the time you eat. It's about the total protein you eat and not how it's spread uniformly throughout the day.

There are even a ton of myths about why you shouldn't fast. Fasting can trigger starvation. Nope, starvation only occurs in situations where no food is eaten over a long period of time. Intermittent fasting should never last that long, as, after 48 hours, your metabolism will start to slow. Short durations of fasting can help boost metabolism and release norepinephrine. This neuro-transmitter-hormone aids in boosting your metabolism and triggers fat burning.

Fasting doesn't break down muscles as fuel, as this only occurs in extreme starvation situations, which intermittent fasting is not. The release of human growth hormone (HGH) protects the muscles from being targeted by gluconeogenesis.

Fasting can be stressful. So is living, and fasting over a short time, doesn't add more stress than getting some exercise. Frequent, short fasting can maintain cortisol levels, which in turn, can regulate your immune system, help you keep a healthy blood pressure, and increase fat metabolism. You won't lose your focus when fasting over a short time. It can improve cognitive function, resulting in learning quicker, and better retention of information.

When coupled with a healthy diet, fasting doesn't force you to overeat. Even if you overeat by a few calories, the total calories consumed for the day is still less as you have skipped a meal or two. Fasting isn't bad for you. Many studies show an array of benefits including an increase in brain-derived neurotrophic factor (BDNF), improves insulin resistance and decreases inflammation.

Then there is the myth that fasting works because your body doesn't process food at night. I have no idea how this myth developed, but if you eat food, your body will digest it, albeit slower while you're asleep, but it's recommended that you don't eat for 2 hours before bedtime. Once there is no more energy from what you have digested, your body will move on to getting energy from glycogen and your body fat.

These aren't even all the myths surrounding a healthy diet and fasting. Now that the fake news is out of the way, let's look at the advantages of intermittent fasting.

ADVANTAGES

Now that we've tackled the misinformation, we can concentrate on the advantages of trying fasting. Why people try new lifestyles and diets is to drop the excess belly fat. With intermittent fasting, you are consuming fewer meals and fewer calories. Your body is forced to digest stored fat to fuel, assisted by HGH and norepinephrine. By keeping to short-term fasting, you can lower your weight easier than trying calorie-restrictive, keto, or paleo diets, which are difficult to follow.

While for most people the external changes are the most important, it's the internal changes that benefit you the most. Animal studies using mice, rats, and fruit flies, have all shown signs of an increase in their life-span when placed on a fasting regime. Although there are yet to be human studies that prove this, fasting is known to improve body conditions leading to longer, healthier lives.

The brain drives our bodies, and when it is bombarded with inflammation, high blood sugar, and free radicals, it can't perform at its optimum. During a fast, there is an increase in BDNF, which is known to fight against depression, neurodegenerative disease, and grow new neurons. Fasting every other day can even help increase long-term memory.

Our joints are also affected by inflammation. This inflammation can cause damage and pain to the joints, making them difficult to move. As soon as the inflammation diminishes, so does the pain, allowing for better movement.

Free radicals occur naturally when oxygen is used to generate energy, resulting in oxidative stress. Oxidative stress can cause chronic diseases while the free radicals damage proteins and DNA. While it's encouraged to eat foods high in antioxidants, fasting can help enhance the body's resistance to oxidative stress.

This brings us to chronic diseases such as high blood pressure, cardiovascular disease, and cholesterol. As it takes nutrient-rich food to get through a fast, you are less likely to consume junk food with many additives that can cause high blood pressure. Limiting these foods during a fast can lower the systolic (upper number) pressure. However, it's important not to fall back on poor eating habits as this will cause your blood pressure to increase again.

Studies have shown that using intermittent fasting can lower your total and LDL—which is considered the "bad"—cholesterol. This in turn helps to protect your heart, but this isn't the only way intermittent fasting can aid it. During a fast, your blood pressure is lower, and there are fewer blood triglycerides, and less blood sugar, all resulting in a healthier environment for your heart. Some animal studies have shown a decrease in inflammatory markers, so this is a good sign for humans too.

Cancer is another chronic disease. It is caused by cells that suddenly start dividing uncontrollably. Animal studies have shown fasting may delay or even block tumor formation, preventing it from adapting and spreading. While human studies still need to be completed, it is known that fasting can help reduce the side effects experienced during chemotherapy.

Autophagy may be another way your body can prevent cancer from starting. This process is the body's way of cleaning up cellular waste such as dysfunctional or broken proteins in damaged cells. By fasting, autophagy starts as soon as glycogen is nearly depleted in the liver.

You can also expect changes to your hormonal levels. Many hormones change during a fast, but the two most important are HGH and insulin. There is a drastic increase in HGH and a decrease in insulin while fasting. The HGH has many functions to benefit health, such as increased fat burning and muscle protection during fasting.

Type 2 diabetes is a global problem due to poor eating habits, low activity, and insulin resistance. During a fast, there is less insulin being secreted as the blood sugar levels drop. In time, this allows cells to become insulin sensitive again as they aren't bombarded by insulin all the time. By fasting, people who suffer from prediabetes (insulin resistance) will prevent themselves from worsening and reduce the risk of type 2 diabetes.

DISADVANTAGES

As simple as fasting may be, it can be a little tough for some people. However, with some help, planning, and foresight, they can achieve their goal of fasting. So don't be put off, it's better to have all the facts, before you start:

Eating disorders

- The restrictiveness of when they may eat can trigger eating disorders in people who have struggled with eating problems in the past.
- People who are or have been treated for eating disorders should avoid fasting; unless under the guidance of their physician.

Digestive problems

- Digestive issues, such as irritable bowel syndrome (IBS), can be exacerbated by intermittent fasting—especially during extended fasts.
- Eating after a fast can cause more stress on an already stressed digestive system, resulting in bloat, constipation, and even indigestion.
- It may be possible to fast for short durations with well-balanced nutrient-rich foods.

Pregnant or breastfeeding

- When pregnant, the body requires more calories than normal. When this isn't provided, it can threaten the baby's development.

- It's advised that women who are breastfeeding or pregnant skip fasting altogether.

Weak immune system

- Anyone considered frail due to surgery, illness, suffering from cancer, etc., shouldn't fast too extremely, as the body needs an adequate number of calories, shorter fasts are better here.
- Fasting can restrict the calories needed and prolong healing.
- Fasting does have some benefits for people going through chemotherapy but should be done under the guidance of a physician.

Adherence issues

- Adhering to a fasting technique can be difficult and comes down to willpower. If you cannot adhere to an eating schedule, then intermittent fasting might not be for you. However, this can be overcome by practicing intermittent fasting a few times a week until you get the hang of it.
- Over-adherence is just as bad as it can cause an obsession with food and lead to binge eating more calories than you should during the eating phase.

Blood sugar issues

- Anyone with diabetes who requires medication or insulin should be wary of trying intermittent fasting.
- As you fast, your blood sugar drops. When it drops too low, it can become dangerous. This is why most diabetics eat frequent meals. Something which you shouldn't do while fasting.
- People with diabetes should work closely with their doctors to find the right balance if they want to try fasting.

Lifestyle

- An inconsistent schedule may be difficult to manage most of the fasting techniques.
- This is particularly bad for those that switch between night and day shifts.
- With some planning and meal preparation in advance, it's possible to give fasting a try.

Medication

- Most medicines should be taken with a meal to avoid possible side effects such as nausea, vomiting, and headaches. When medications are time sensitive, this will have an impact on whether intermittent fasting is possible or not.

- You may have to schedule meals when you need to take your medication.

Focus and concentration

- Extended fasts can cause a loss of focus and the inability to concentrate—especially if you can only think about food.
- The best course of action is to ease into the fast and choose one that best suits your work. Practicing the fast will make it easier to deal with the thoughts of food.
- Some people may have clarity while fasting, while others don't. You won't know if this affects you or not until you try.

Intensive training

- High-intensity training requires a lot of glucose, which isn't readily available when fasting for extended periods.
- Fasts should be scheduled to allow the person training to eat before and after the session to keep their muscles fueled.

- Building muscle also poses a problem when fasting, as it requires ample protein to be available to be successful.
- When training intensively, a specific training schedule and diet may be required while fasting.

Sleep problems

- People who already suffer from sleeping problems may find fasting adds more problems when they go to sleep hungry. This can be avoided by changing your fasting period.
- A meal should be consumed before going to sleep, as this will lower disruptions to sleeping patterns.

Anyone who is underweight should also avoid fasting, as they need enough calories to increase their weight to a healthier level. In some cases, fasting is possible for those who generally wouldn't be able to. However, it's important to seek advice from your physician.

Possible Side Effects

Intermittent fasting isn't inherently dangerous, but it is wise to be cautious when trying it the first time. There is no scientific data to prove or disprove the benefits of fasting for a long time, as most studies have been completed on animals. However, there are a slew of side effects you may experience. Luckily though, they are easily managed:

Hunger and cravings

- You will feel hungry and have a rumbling tummy.
- You may suffer from binging and overeating.
- Luckily this can be managed with the preparation of well-balanced meals.

Digestive issues

- Due to dietary changes, there is a chance of constipation—especially when not enough water is drunk.
- These changes may also result in extensive bouts of diarrhea and bloat.
- This side effect can be overcome with nutrient-dense food before and after a fast.

Mood changes

- The stress of not eating may cause an increase in cortisol, leading to cravings and hunger.

- You may experience mood shifts resulting in irritability, anxiety, and possibly depression. Hangry is a real emotion.
- These changes are due to lowered blood sugar and are very common.
- Add mood-enhancing foods such as fish, nuts, seeds, and oats to help manage these feelings.
- Once overcome, you will be filled with a sense of pride in accomplishing your goal.

Fatigue

- The lower the blood sugar, the less energy you will have. You may even have disturbed sleep, such as trying to fall asleep or staying asleep.
- Metabolizing fat results in a lot of salt and water waste, meaning you may have to get up in the middle of the night.
- Luckily, this is temporary and will likely only last a few days as most of your glycogen is used.

Bad breath

- Acetone is a type of ketone which is expelled through the mouth, resulting in a sickly-sweet smell.

- Dehydration will lead to a dry mouth, causing bad-breath bacteria to multiply and create a stink.
- Chewing on some gum and brushing your teeth after meals will reduce the smell.

Dehydration

- Many people suffer from dehydration as they forget to drink water. As meals that contain liquid are skipped, this can cause dehydration to worsen. As this gets worse, constipation can occur.
- Always keep a full water bottle handy. The only downside to drinking water is the frequent bathroom trips. Keep an eye on your urine color, as this will tell you if you're dehydrated or not.

Other

- There is a possibility of suffering from nausea, headaches, or dizziness due to low blood sugar.
- Fasting headaches are generally found in the front of the head and can vary from mild to moderate.

- This passes in time as your blood sugar stabilizes. It may also be a side effect of caffeine withdrawal. Remember, you can have coffee during a fast, just none of the additives such as milk or sugar.
- Be wary of drinking alcohol after a fast. Alcohol on an empty stomach can cause you to get drunk faster than expected. Always have at least a snack before drinking.

Long-term

- You may develop an unhealthy obsession with getting the correct number of calories and nutrients.
- Some people can't maintain healthy eating as they keep exceeding calorie intake.
- There is a possibility of fertility issues when experiencing an irregular menstrual cycle. If a period slows or stops, end your fast.
- There is the potential to lose hair if you don't eat enough protein or vitamin B.
- All of these negative side effects can be avoided with a well-balanced and nutrient-dense eating plan that gives you all the nutrients and calories you need.

All diets and lifestyle changes will have side effects until you are used to them. It can take up to a month to fully adapt to fasting. Remember that intermittent fasting will put a strain on your body. With some fasting practice, most of the side effects can be overcome.

Despite learning the truth behind the myths, you may still have questions. Let's start with the obvious one. Is intermittent fasting starvation? Starvation is the abscess of food, while intermittent fasting is the absence of food for a set period. Binging and overeating are common problems when it comes to people who fast for the first time. Sometimes it's difficult to know what you're supposed to eat after a fast—especially when your stomach is demanding a meal. The best possible meal you can eat is one with lean proteins, low glycemic index (low GI) carbohydrates, and good fats, in the ratio of 30:40:30. Ensure the foods you choose are nutrient-dense as this will help your gut.

SUCCESS STORY

To show how easy intermittent fasting is, let's review the success Kariss Grimm had. Kariss is a mom of two rowdy boys and is a military wife. In November 2018, she wasn't happy with how she looked and set herself the goals of losing weight and getting stronger. She settled on trying intermittent fasting and prepared herself to try the 16:8 technique.

This was successful for her, as she was able to eat what she craved within eight hours and still had the energy to walk every day. She continued with this technique until she lost 70 pounds. One day she got too busy to eat her usual number of meals and ended up only eating a single, large meal. Realizing this suited her lifestyle better, she switched from 16:8 to the One Meal a Day (OMAD) for another year. Over time, the way she ate no longer felt like a diet but a new lifestyle.

Kariss dropped 125 pounds before getting a trainer to help her with weight-lifting techniques. She even had the time to take up martial arts, though she still walks on the days she isn't in the gym. As she adapted to OMAD, her body told her what foods were needed to fuel her, and she never felt the need to eat outside her one meal. Even if she does, she can easily return to eating a single meal the following day. She truly is an intermittent-fasting inspiration to us all.

STARTING INTERMITTENT FASTING: BALANCING MASTER HORMONES

In the previous chapter, we looked at the hormones that play a role during fasting, now it's time to look at what regulates them. In your brain, there is the hypothalamus and the pituitary gland. Together, they work to become the central command of the brain that controls all vital bodily functions through hormones.

The hypothalamus communicates with the pituitary gland with hormones such as dopamine and somatostatin. These hormones tell the gland what it should make and secrete. This is the heart of the endocrine system. This combo is in charge of growth, sexual development, plus regulates almost all of your bodily functions. Without them, the body's functions go unregulated. Anyone who suffers damage to the pituitary will have to remain on hormone replacement medication—dependent on what isn't being secreted—for the rest of their life.

The pituitary gland is divided into two sections, the anterior (front) and posterior (back) lobes. Each section is in charge of secreting specific hormones that fulfill different tasks.

The anterior lobe produces HGH, thyroid-stimulating hormone (TSH), adrenocorticotropic hormone (ATCH), follicle-stimulating hormone (FSH), luteinizing hormone (LH), and prolactin.

In children, HGH helps them grow, while in adults, it aids in maintaining healthy bones and muscles. The hormones FSH and LH are gonadotropic hormones. The stimulation of sperm production in men, the stimulation of ovaries to make estrogen, and egg development in women are governed by FSH. Meanwhile, LH stimulates ovulation and testosterone production. Prolactin can affect fertility and aid in milk production, but it isn't only produced in women. Men with high prolactin will struggle with erectile dysfunction and a lower sex drive.

Thyroid-stimulating hormone is in charge of getting the thyroid to make thyroid hormones. Thyroid hormones manage the metabolism, the nervous system, and energy levels. Adrenocorticotropic hormone helps you respond to stress by stimulating the adrenal glands to secrete cortisol.

The posterior lobe secretes the hormones vasopressin and oxytocin. Vasopressin—also known as antidiuretic hormone (ADH)—is responsible for the water and salt balance in the body. It also aids in increasing water absorption and blood pressure. It is made in the hypothalamus and stored in the pituitary gland until needed. Oxytocin in women stimulates the release of milk and contracts the uterus during childbirth. In men, this hormone aids with ejaculation and sperm production.

The pituitary is considered the master gland in your body because its control of these hormones will influence what happens to you when you are fasting. Once you start fasting, there is a change in the endocrine responses, resulting in lower oxidative stress, and an increase in insulin sensitivity and metabolism. As long as your fasting sessions are kept short, the pituitary won't cause your body to enter fat-storing mode.

There is also a change at the hypothalamus-pituitary-thyroid axis which is in charge of regulating metabolism and stress response. Because of this, your leptin sensitivity increases, and you react better to the appetite reducer. This is your body's way of saving energy where it can.

As mentioned earlier, women tend to store fat better than using it, likely as the body's way of preserving reproductive function. Luckily, due to fasting, the pituitary starts secreting more HGH, which increases fat metabolism. Even if you aren't committed to fasting quite yet, know that HGH decreases as you age, resulting in weakening bone density and muscle strength. Even fasting a few times a week can help bolster HGH to prevent this.

Now, for what you have all been waiting for, let's learn more about the different ways you can intermittently fast.

Weaknesses are just strengths in the wrong environment.

— MARIANNE CANTWELL

4

TYPES OF INTERMITTENT FASTING

How a person chooses their way of intermittent fasting is up to them. However, the fasting technique you decide on should match your activity level, lifestyle, and what you can adhere to. Never push yourself to a point where you feel ill.

SHORT-TERM FASTING

Fasting techniques can be short or long-term fasts. If you are new to intermittent fasting, start with a short-term fast, then build up your adherence to the longer fasts.

Spontaneous Meal Skipping

If you're not ready to commit yourself to intermittent fasting quite yet then consider spontaneously skipping a meal now and again. Why eat any meal if you aren't hungry? If you do feel hungry later in the day and it's not time for your next meal, you can tide yourself over with water or zero-calorie drinks. This way, you eat 500–1,000 calories less a week. It's an easy way to lose about half a pound a month and ease your way into fasting with fewer side effects and little planning.

Circadian Rhythm Eating

This fasting technique is also known as the sun cycle diet, as you're encouraged to only eat during the daytime and fast during the night. This fasting method matches our internal waking and sleep clock, which is controlled by the hypothalamus. When you're exposed to light, this signals you to wake up, while the absence of light will prepare you to wind down for the day. As you wake, your adrenal glands secrete cortisol, which peaks later in the afternoon, before it starts to diminish in the later part of the afternoon and evening. A lower level of cortisol can affect your metabolism. This coupled with meals later in the night—which causes a spike in insulin—could disturb your sleep.

There is no limitation on what you can eat, and this diet can easily be coupled with exercise. However, it can be difficult to maintain—especially with social outings in the evening.

People who follow this technique will get up earlier in the day to eat, but stop eating when it reaches six or seven in the evening. The idea behind this technique is that you fuel yourself for the day's activities, but you aren't that active at night, so there is no need to eat.

Although this seems similar to intermittent fasting, it isn't quite the same, as you don't get to choose when you want to eat your meals. For this reason, it may be difficult for night-shift workers to get benefits from this way of eating. For those who like to start your day as soon as the sun comes up, go outside and spend about five minutes enjoying the sunrise before getting breakfast started.

16:8 Technique

This is the fasting technique most people like to start with and the one I adhere to now for most of the time, although I do switch to 18:6 for a few days a week. You fast for 16 hours, followed by an 8-hour eating window. When you fast and when you eat is up to you. Most people like to fast from 8 p.m. to noon, as I do, but you can tweak this to suit your needs. Just ensure that you don't eat two hours before going to sleep.

As long as you are avoiding processed foods and consuming whole foods, this technique can be done a few days out of the week until you are ready to dedicate yourself to it. To avoid feeling hungry, remain well hydrated, and busy yourself with chores, work, or even meditation to get through any hunger pangs that may arise. If you're struggling, try cinnamon tea to help suppress your hunger.

18:6 Technique

If you find the 16:8 technique too easy and want to ramp up the fat burning in your body, consider trying the 18:6. You only need to last without food for two more hours. Plenty of time to eat two main meals and possibly a snack. With this technique, you are switching from glucose to ketones as an energy source, and you may get a little tired. It's a good idea to try and get some extra rest, if you can, and more hydration to see yourself through the fasting period.

Schedule fasting in such a way that your day isn't negatively affected. Any food you eat now should include lean proteins, vegetables, fruit, and complex carbohydrates. Avoid eating any saturated or trans fats and refined carbs. Don't forget to include your mono- and polyunsaturated fats to help bolster metabolism.

You may find that you'll lose a lot of fluid, which should be replaced, or you will become dehydrated. As long as your drink has no calories, you can go wild with ideas. Add black coffee and tea to your list, but don't forget herbal teas, which can also suppress feelings of hunger. Although you may not need to supplement minerals and vitamins with this technique.

The Fast Diet

Known as the 5:2 technique, this isn't considered a true fasting technique by some. When starting this diet, you get to eat normally for five days, and on two non-sequential days, you should eat roughly a quarter of your usual calorie allowance. For women, roughly 500 calories should be consumed during the two days of fasting. How this diet differs from a standard fast, is that there is no time control over when you eat, as you eat every day. However, this will depend on how you break up the 500 calories.

It's important to budget your calories appropriately and ensure you get enough nutrients to make it through the day. As long as you only eat 500 calories, you can have as many meals as you wish. You want to aim for nutri-ent-rich foods, but don't discredit soups. Bone broth is an excellent source of minerals and nutrients, keeps you hydrated, plus it's low in calories.

The five days that you get to eat normally shouldn't be considered cheat days. You are creating a calorie deficit, and it's pointless to go through this technique if you're going to overeat the rest of the time. Meals, especially those during the day before the fasting day, should be well-balanced, with everything you may need to get through the fast in relative comfort. Technically no food is off limits when you try the 5:2 technique, the main concern is to remain in a calorie deficit.

This can be a tough technique to attempt if you haven't done intermittent fasting before. Take the time to train yourself, as this will help you avoid overeating on your non-fasting days. If you're trying it, and you find your fasting days too difficult, consider placing them in the week on days you know you won't be very active. Alternatively, consider distractions such as reading, walking, and drinking zero-calorie drinks.

LONG-TERM FASTING

Long-term fasting is any fasting technique that lasts 20 hours or more. Prolonged or extensive fasting is anything that extends beyond 24 hours and may not work for everyone, nor should it be done often.

Warrior Diet

This is where the fasting techniques get a little tougher to adhere to. The Warrior Diet allows for an eating period of 4 hours and a fasting period of 20. Specific exercises can be done while on this diet, but only once you have made this your new lifestyle. This diet is said to mimic the life of the nomadic hunter-gatherers as they would spend all day hunting and looking for food, only spend a short time eating what they caught.

There are no food restrictions. However, it may be difficult to try and eat 2,000 calories within four hours. Aim to eat about 90% of what you need and spread it across the four hours or as a single meal. Stick to eating unprocessed foods, as these will provide more benefits to your body. You can even enjoy some wine with or after dinner as this helps with protein digestion. Although binge eating can occur while on this fast, it's rare that people overeat if they stick to well-balanced, pre-prepared meals and avoid poor fats and refined sugars.

During the fasting phase of this technique, low-calorie meals are allowed to aid in keeping energy levels up. However, these aren't meals but rather snacking options such as small amounts of yogurt, some berries, or even soup to keep you going until the feeding period. If you want to fast fully for 20 hours, don't eat anything.

However, keep in mind, as a woman, this can have negative effects. During long fasts, the hormones luteinizing and FSH are lower, which can impact bone health, ovary size, and fertility rates in women.

One Meal a Day (OMAD)

This is pretty self-explanatory. You have about an hour to eat a meal, and then you fast for the rest of the day. While some women handle this fast with no problem, others may find it too difficult to maintain for a long time. There is no need to switch to this lifestyle if it's too difficult. Try 1–2 days a week with OMAD and spend the rest of the time on the 16:8 technique. This is the upgrade to the Warrior Diet, and you get to choose whenever to have your meal.

The biggest challenge with this technique is deciding what you are going to eat. Meals need to be high in nutrients and calories to make up for not eating the rest of the time. This likely means you won't be getting all the calories you need. At the very least, you should eat about 1,200 calories to maintain energy levels and meet most of your nutritional needs. It may be a good idea to practice meal prep, so you can ensure you are getting everything you need to fuel yourself for the next day.

This requires a lot of willpower and discipline but will suit a busy lifestyle for someone who only has time to eat a single meal. By eating this way, you give your digestive tract a break, but it will have an impact on athletes that do intense training. Ensure you are eating cooked meals, so they are easy to digest.

Eat Stop Eat: The 24-Hour Fast

This technique is when you fast for 24 hours, followed by a regular eating thereafter. It's advised to only attempt this once or twice a week. Most people have never known a day without food, and you'll have your belly and brain playing tricks on you. One day of no food won't cause irreparable damage to you, even though it may feel that way if this is your first time. Ease into this technique by eating well the day before the fast. Concentrate on food that makes you feel fuller for longer, such as protein and high-fiber vegetables.

After 24 hours of not eating, expect your stomach to have shrunk a little. Don't force a large meal, as this will cause digestive issues. Make a small portion of cooked food—steamed veggies or oatmeal—and eat it to allow a gentle break from your fast. If you are still hungry, wait about an hour before having a regular meal.

Schedule your fasting days in the week for when you don't have to be very active so that you can get as much rest as possible. This technique can be combined with weight training on days that you are refueling your body. Remember that the idea behind this technique is to allow for a deficit of calories across the entire week. Don't overeat after breaking your fast.

Alternate-Day Fasting

With this technique, fasting lasts for 24 hours, then eating normally for another 24 hours. This is similar to the 5:2, but instead of 1–2 days, you keep the pattern of 24 hours fasting and eating. This can be tough, so be prepared to feel very hungry when you fast, and prepare well-balanced meals on your eating days.

If this seems out of reach, follow a similar eating pattern as seen in the 5:2 technique. On the days you would normally fast, allow yourself to consume 25–40% of your usual calories (500–700), concentrating on proteins and fiber-rich foods to help you feel full. As you find the alternating fasting days becoming easier, lower the number of calories you eat until you no longer eat any.

There will be hunger, and you may feel as if you are starving, but you aren't. Stay hydrated, supplement if you need it, and don't forget about adding salt, and drinking electrolytes. Even though you think you aren't dehydrated, because you're drinking water, you are losing essential salts, which can lead to dehydration. Keep yourself busy, so that hunger doesn't distract you.

Prolonged Fasting

Most prolonged fasting can last up to 36 hours but can be as long as 72 or more. The point of prolonged fasting is to make use of the fat-burning metabolism and autophagy to detox yourself. This is not something you should jump into on your first day of fasting. It can take months of practice to get to this point.

The best way to handle long fasts is to have your last meal in the evening. That way, most of the fasting period will be during the night while you sleep. Although some people like to attempt a dry fast, it isn't recommended, so be sure to drink plenty of fluids and electrolytes (magnesium, potassium, sodium, and calcium) to keep your body running well.

The best way to tackle prolonged fasting is to prepare yourself for the main event. Have a cooked meal prepared and waiting for you by the end of the fast. Start with a small, easily digestible meal to break your fast, then have a larger meal after an hour. This allows your digestive tract to wake up and start digesting before you give it more difficult foods to break down. Once the fast is over, you can continue a 16:8 fast if you wish to keep up with all the benefits of fasting.

This technique takes a lot of dedication, and you may have to turn down social events or schedule your fast around them. Only plan prolonged fasts a few times a year, as it may influence your hormones. If you feel unwell or the side effects can't be overcome, break your fast. You can always try again at a future date. Slowly extend fasting times as you train your body for a prolonged fast.

CELEBRITY FASTING SUCCESS

Kourtney Kardashian is a household name, and many people know about her way of life. However, did you know that she is an advocate of intermittent fasting? Kourtney generally likes to stop eating at 7 p.m. and will fast for roughly 14–16 hours before eating again. In the past, she combined the ketogenic diet with fasting, but now only uses fasting as it's less complicated.

The only thing she considers as a cheat on fasting is that she takes a collagen drink before bed. Yet this seems to barely break her fast, as she remains steadfast in not eating until after her morning training session, somewhere between 10 and 11 a.m. On top of the 14–16 hour fast, she will do a 24-hour fast once a week to help detox her body.

To prevent the 24-hour fast from being too tough, her meals before the fast contain salads high in fiber, avocado smoothies, and meals without grains and legumes, as she prefers vegetables. During the 24-hour fast, Kourtney will only drink bone broth, water, black coffee (to boost metabolism), and green tea. She keeps herself busy, as this prevents her thoughts from being consumed by hunger.

While training herself to do a 24-hour fast, she developed several coping mechanisms to get through it. Firstly, she brushes her teeth, as this signals the end of eating. She also uses an app to track how long her fast is going. Then, when the sugar cravings hit, she beats them back by drinking her water with lemon slices or a touch of apple cider vinegar, or a cup of hot green tea. If she can fast with her busy life, so can you!

STARTING INTERMITTENT FASTING: SUPPLEMENTING WHILE FASTING

While attempting a short-term fast, there shouldn't be any need to take supplements when you have a balanced diet. Supplements should only be taken when you have a deficiency in a mineral or vitamin. Taking too much of a supplement can be just as detrimental to your health as having a deficiency. Before you take a supplement, talk to your doctor. They will likely be able to give you advice on the best supplements you may need—especially if you plan to exercise.

However, if you are trying prolonged fasts that last longer than 24 hours, you'll need to take a few supplements. When going through a fast, the body consumes everything it has to spare, and now needs replacements of various minerals and vitamins. If these aren't replaced, side effects will become more severe. When taking supplements, some will break a fast while others won't. If you need a supplement that may break your fast, take it when it's time to eat, and take non-fast-breaking supplements whenever you need them. Here are a few supplements you may need that won't break your fast:

Collagen

- Pure collagen can be taken without breaking your fast.
- It is needed to maintain the elasticity, strength, and hydration of your skin.
- Collagen may affect how efficient autophagy is.

Creatine

- Creatine helps to strengthen lean muscles and aids in recovery.

Electrolytes

- Sodium is required to avoid headaches and muscle cramps.
- Potassium helps improve heart health and boosts energy.
- Calcium helps bones retain strength.

L-tyrosine

- L-tyrosine helps to boost mood, manage stress, and aid muscle recovery.

Probiotics

- There are many products you can use, but not all can be taken on an empty stomach. Ensure you read the label of the product you use to be sure.
- Probiotics improve gut health.

Water-soluble vitamins

- These vitamins are excreted out of the body through urine and not stored.
- Vitamin C helps heal the body and is an antioxidant.

- Vitamin B-complex may cause nausea in some people when taken on an empty stomach. These vitamins play a vital role in making enzymes and helping carbohydrate metabolism.
- Folic acid is needed to make and maintain cells, playing a role in preventing cancer.

Here are a few more supplements you may need but should be taken with food, as they can break your fast:

Amino acids

- Amino acids such as L-glutamine and branched-chain amino acids (BCAA) should be supplemented while fasting.
- Amino acids are used to build proteins, repair tissue damage, and aid in nutrient absorption.

Fat-soluble vitamins

- Fat-soluble vitamins include A, D, E, and K, and are stored in fat molecules.
- These vitamins aid in growth, normal function in the body, and maintenance of tissues.

Curcumin

- Curcumin helps to improve heart health, prevents certain cancers, lowers the risk of Alzheimer's, and lowers insulin resistance.

Omega-3 fatty acid

- This fatty acid helps to lower the risks of cardiovascular disease.

Chromium and vanadium

- These minerals help maintain healthy blood sugar levels.

Magnesium

- This mineral and electrolyte support nerve and muscle function and aids energy production.

Zinc

- This trace mineral increases nerve communication and regulates hormones.

Copper

- This trace mineral helps to make melanin used to protect you from the sun's rays.

Iodine

- Iodine helps to make thyroid hormone.

Medium-chain triglycerides (MCT)

- Although you may not need it, these healthy fats will help you stay in fat metabolism for longer.

Soluble fiber

- This type of fiber will help you feel fuller for longer and keep you regular.

Listen to your body during the extended fasting period. If you feel you need to eat a certain type of food, there is likely something in that food your body needs. In the next chapter, we will look at what you should and shouldn't do while on a fast.

Real change, enduring change, happens one step at a time.

— RUTH BADER GINSBURG

5

DOS AND DON'TS OF FASTING

Regardless of which fasting technique you want to try, there are some pitfalls you need to be wary of. Once you know what potential problems you may face, they will be significantly easier to overcome.

WHAT TO AVOID

The first aspect of fasting you need to face is hunger. People handle hunger in different ways, but one of the most detrimental to your health is to overeat. After not having food for some time, you may feel you need to eat as much as possible in a short duration. There is no point in fasting if you are going to overeat. To avoid this happening, be mindful of how you eat the foods you use to break your fast. Prepare smaller portions and take your time chewing them instead of wolfing down your food. It takes time for your stomach to signal to your brain that it's starting to get full.

Caffeine and zero-calorie sodas are a great way to trick your stomach into thinking you're full. However, you need to be sure of what sweetener the zero-calorie drink is using, as some sweeteners may contain dextrose (a type of sugar), which will cause an insulin response and break your fast. For this reason, I don't drink them before 12 p.m. However, don't push your fast for too long, as an extensive fast isn't good for you. Long-term fasts without preparation will cause binging, overeating, increased side effects. This can cause people to quit because they feel intermittent fasting is not working for them, as they are not seeing the results they hoped for.

When you feel extreme hunger, you should consider why. Are you fasting too long? Have you had enough protein during your previous meal? Are you having caffeine withdrawal? Each of these can play a role in you feeling hungrier than you really are.

There is no need to quit caffeine; just what you add to it. Coffee and tea are encouraged during fasting as they fill your tummy, and the heat is a great comfort.

During your eating period, it's wise to add some protein to every meal with high-fiber vegetables. The combination of protein and fiber allows you to feel fuller for longer, beating back those hunger pangs.

Many people who start fasting for the first time fail to hydrate themselves adequately, causing them to experience more side effects than necessary. Even when they're eating, they fail to get enough moisture in their food. When planning a fast, ensure it is full of low-sugar fruit, vegetables, water, and electrolytes to fuel you. Then when you fast, be sure to drink more than enough water—for some people, this can be as much as half a gallon extra than they usually drink.

You will also need to realize that any intensive training will be affected by a change in diet. The sessions need to be powered one way or another. Depending on what kind of training you want to do, this will determine when you refuel yourself.

Finally, and probably what sets most people back on a diet, is quitting when you make a mistake. Fasting takes time to get used to, so be prepared to stumble now and again. This isn't a failure, but rather an opportunity to learn from it. Try again to do better tomorrow and adjust how you fast.

BEST FOODS TO FUEL A FAST

Your fast is only as good as the foods you have eaten to fuel your body. The worse the food you put into yourself, the worse your fast will be. Here are some examples of foods you can eat when you start to fast:

Protein

- Protein powders (pea and whey) for extra amino acids, legumes, nuts, eggs, steak, pork chops, chicken thighs, cottage cheese, and seitan (avoid if you're gluten intolerant).
- Eat red meat in smaller quantities than lean pork and poultry.

Probiotics

- Unsweetened yogurt, kefir, kimchi, and pickled vegetables.

Healthy fats

- Oils (olive, avocado, coconut, and MCT), ghee, avocados, nuts, and different nut butters (sugar-free), olives, flax seeds, and chia seeds.
- Avoid store-bought salad dressings and make your own.

Fish and seafood

- Wild caught salmon, cod, rainbow trout, mackerel, sardines, anchovies, mussels, oysters, crab, lobster, and shrimp.

Vegetables

- Spinach, chard, arugula, kale, broccoli, cauliflower, Brussels sprouts, cabbage, celery, asparagus, and seaweed.
- Potatoes can be eaten with or without their skin, hot or cold. However, when a potato is eaten after it's been cooked and allowed to fully cool, they form resistant starch. This starch makes a great fuel for you and your gut bacteria.

Fruits

- Aim to eat fruits that are nutrient-rich and with low to medium-sugar content.
- Strawberries, raspberries, blackberries, kiwi, grapefruit, apples, lemons, limes, avocado, tomatoes, blueberries, and papaya.

Dairy

- Get vitamin D-fortified milk, as this will help to absorb the calcium easier and help build strong bones.

Whole grains

- Oatmeal, millet, quinoa, and rice (wild, black, or brown).

Legumes

- Beans (black, green, lima, and kidney), lentils, chickpeas (garbanzo beans), and soybeans.
- If you miss having dips, use chickpeas to make fresh hummus whenever you want.

Herbs and spices

- Many herbs and spices have anti-inflammatory effects that can be added to your food.
- Cinnamon, cloves, turmeric, ginger, sage, rosemary, thyme, and whatever else suits your taste.

Remember that you won't get the same quantity of food during a fast, so you need to look at the quality of what you'll eat.

BEST DRINKS DURING A FAST

Unless you are a purist with fasting, you don't have to only stick to water. There are many different drinks you can enjoy during your fasting period. Plain water can get a little boring after a time, so spice it up with some cucumber or lemon slices. You can also use 1–2 tablespoons of apple cider vinegar in water to help suppress feelings of hunger. Alternatively, soda water or warm water help keep your stomach full and adequately hydrated.

Many people enjoy zero-calorie drinks as a way to suppress their hunger. However, be warned that many of these drinks can still cause an insulin response due to the sweeteners used. Read labels carefully to see what sweeteners are in the drinks. Anything with stevia, monk fruit, and erythritol should be fine but use these sweeteners sparingly.

Drink black coffee and tea, as well as herbal teas (as long as they don't have fruit in them,) as often as you want. They are full of antioxidants, boost metabolism, and help keep you warm and comfortable. Another warm drink you can consider is bone or vegetable broth. These are easily made at home, are low in calories, and are high in vitamins, minerals, and electrolytes. It makes for a perfect snack if you need to overcome a few more hours on a fast.

When the hunger gets too much, but you don't want to eat, you can consider having a bulletproof coffee or tea. Yes, this breaks your eating fast, but you will remain in ketosis, and your autophagy will continue as if you hadn't broken your fast. Bulletproof drinks are warm drinks that contain fat—such as ghee, MCT, coconut oil, or butter—which will drive back your hunger and satisfy you, without causing an insulin spike.

While alcohol (limited), smoothies, and protein shakes are fine to drink while you're eating, they should be avoided during a fast.

MANAGING HUNGER

When you start to fast, hunger will always be at the back of your mind. You'll need to manage and overcome it to get through your fasting period. Luckily, there are many ways for you to achieve this!

Before starting your fasting lifestyle, begin by cutting out unnecessary foods—such as processed foods or foods high in carbohydrates—and increase the good quality fats in your diet. Include moderate protein in this and your body will be more prepared for what it'll face. You'll also need to cut back on alcohol consumption.

Hunger can be triggered by poor sleep and stress. Improve sleep by looking at your sleep hygiene. Do this by ensuring your bedroom has no distractions, is cool and well ventilated, shielded from most noise and light, and you don't exercise or eat within 2–3 hours of going to sleep. Combating stress is different for each person. Some like exercise, others do yoga or read a book. Take the time to figure out how you can combat stress in your life and start doing it!

Your main defense against hunger is hydration, and not just using water. Warm drinks such as bone broth or bulletproof coffee can keep you in ketosis and autophagy, and fill the belly. These drinks will also help with keeping your electrolytes in balance without the need to supplement.

Change the way you think about your fast. If you're sitting doing nothing and only thinking about when the fast will end, it's going to be unbearable! Get busy with light exercise, housework, hobbies, anything to keep you from getting bored and thinking about food. While doing these activities, think of all the benefits you are getting from your fasting lifestyle. Guaranteed, this will distract you from the thoughts of food.

If you have an issue with late-night snacking, go to bed earlier. You don't need to go to sleep yet. By brushing your teeth and climbing into bed with a good book, you'll be distracted and not think about food.

Hunger is normal while fasting, but extreme hunger that can't be ignored is a sign that maybe the way you are fasting isn't right for you. Break your fast then review the technique you are trying or drop the duration by a few hours. You're still learning about your body and how you fast. There are bound to be a few slip-ups now and again. Keep going!

HOW TO BREAK A FAST

The first time you break a fast, you may feel that you want a burger, shakes, and fries, but consider how you would feel after eating that. There is nothing wrong with breaking your fast this way if it's comfortable for you. However, you may likely experience digestive distress and overeat later in the day. The meal that breaks your fast should wake your digestive tract gently before you give it tougher food to digest. It's best to aim for foods low in fat, sugar, and raw fiber.

Let's look at drinks you can use to break your fast. Broths, or light soups with protein and easily digested carbohydrates such as legumes, are a great way to end a long fast. Smoothies can also be a gentle wake-up for your stomach. Although there is fiber in the fruit and vegetables used, the blending action breaks up the fiber, making it easier to digest.

A glass of plain water before you eat also wakes your gut up and prevents you from overeating the meal that follows. You can even add some apple cider vinegar to the water.

Meals that break your fast should be at least 500 calories with nutrient-dense protein and fiber. Stick to lean proteins such as fish or poultry. If the meat seems too dense for you to eat, add it to a broth instead. A warm salad containing kale, spinach, broccoli, or cauliflower with a sprinkle of almond shavings or chia seeds makes a welcome meal. A meal without the tough fiber you'd have to digest if you ate the vegetables raw.

If you prefer something with a little more protein, try a hard-boiled egg with avocado or yogurt with a handful of blueberries. These aren't the only fruits you can use to break your fast. Have a small portion of watermelon. It may be high in sugar but it hydrates you well and gives ample fiber. Alternatively, you can have a small banana. This fruit is nutrient-dense and replenishes your body with lost minerals and vitamins. To prevent the sugar content giving you a large sugar boost, have it with some nut butter to slow digestion and absorption of the banana.

SUCCESS STORY

Scott Jennings is a Republican adviser, a CNN political contributor, and a partner at RunSwitch Public Relations. To say the very least, he's a very busy man! However, in January 2019, Scott came to an unpleasant realization when going out to dinner with friends that his suit barely fit him. This wasn't a new problem. He was already well aware that he was physically and emotionally unwell.

Scott had always been a large kid and now, an even larger adult who weighed over 250 pounds and was addicted to sugar. He had tried numerous ways to lose weight, but each time it came back with a vengeance. Scott knew his weight problems came from social pressures, stress, anxiety, and boredom. Until he found a way to bypass them, he wasn't going to get healthier.

Yet, he wouldn't be defeated, so he started researching ways to lose his excess weight and stumbled across intermittent fasting. Once he started, he never looked back. He was not only steadily losing weight, but his body fat was also melting away.

Originally, he started with the 16:8 technique before he eventually settled on OMAD when he eats a single meal, somewhere between 1 p.m. and 5 p.m. Although he never skimps on a meal, he never binges. Once he's full, he stops eating. Occasionally, he reaches a plateau, but thanks to the support from a friend who fasts with him, he's able to overcome it and continue with his new way of life. It just shows that when times get tough, a friend in your corner is a valuable asset.

STARTING INTERMITTENT FASTING: RESTORING REPRODUCTIVE HORMONES, THYROID, AND MELATONIN

As already discussed, with extended fasts, a woman can trigger her body to think that it should be storing fat and stop all attempts at reproduction. This is because extended periods without food can cause havoc on the reproductive hormones. When the reproductive hormones are out of harmony, so are the metabolic hormones, resulting in a change in metabolic function.

When estrogen is disrupted, fertility decreases, causing a change in mood, increases in stress and anxiety, weight fluctuations, and many other factors. When one hormone is out of balance, it can affect other hormones such as cortisol and thyroid hormone. When cortisol is out of balance it can cause:

- lowered energy
- anxiety
- increased sugar cravings
- insomnia

With an imbalance in the thyroid hormone, you're likely to experience:

- increased weight
- anxiety and depression
- dry skin and hair
- irregular periods

This is why no woman should ever do an extended fast without fully training themselves to do it. By giving yourself time to ease into a fast, you are preparing your body to undergo several changes. Warning signs that the fasting technique you have chosen is doing more harm than good include:

- irregular or absent periods
- poor quality sleep
- changes in digestion

- becoming moody or experiencing extended brain fog
- negative changes to the condition of your skin or hair
- feeling cold all the time

Even if you have your period, you need to ensure it's healthy in its frequency, color, and smell, as this may be the first indication that something isn't quite right.

Fasting also seems to improve the quality of sleep as most techniques match our natural circadian rhythms—especially with not eating late into the night. During a fast, there is an increase in HGH and the neurotransmitter orexin, allowing you to wake refreshed and alert after a restful sleep. These changes can occur in as little as a week from starting your fast. So, a fast can aid in waking less during the night, allow you to get more rapid eye movement (REM), lower how much you move while you sleep, and increase how peacefully you sleep.

However, timing your meals is vital, as large meals too close to going to sleep have the opposite effect. Late meals can cause an increase in temperature, possibly upset the belly, and makes it difficult to fall asleep. All these disruptions to your sleep can cause your melatonin to lower, causing even more troubled sleep and possibly resulting in insomnia.

Overcoming Fasting as a Woman

We may be more sensitive to fasting than men, but that doesn't mean we can't get the results we want! We just need to go about it a little more carefully:

- Avoid fasting extensively for consecutive days by spreading them throughout the week.
- Avoid intense training while on a fast.
- Avoid eating large meals within 2–3 hours before going to sleep.
- If you notice too many side effects, change the way you fast.
- Some women find it easier not to fast during their menstrual cycle.
- Review your diet and add foods that bolster hormonal health, such as fatty fish, chicken breasts, and cherries.
- Ease into a fast, and slowly extend it. The more practice you get, the less your hormones will be affected by a sudden change.

Fasting affects the sex hormones of both genders, but as long as the fast is short-term, the reproductive hormones shouldn't change too much. Some preliminary data shows that fasting could be used for hyperandrogenism women with high levels of androgens who have polycystic ovarian syndrome (PCOS) (Cienfuegos et al., 2022). It's believed that while fasting, they could have regular periods and increased fertility. However, more studies need to be completed before this can be proved.

Now that you understand how to fuel your body for a fast, let's see how exercise can influence how a fast will run its course.

Nobody is built like you, you design yourself.

— JAY-Z

6

BENDING YOUR BODY

F asting is but one way to lose the weight you carry. Another is exercise. One of the biggest questions asked by those that start fasting is if they can continue their exercise regimen if they are fasting. The answer may surprise you.

BENEFITS OF EXERCISE

Countless scientific articles are dedicated to the benefits exercise grants us. It isn't just about losing weight and strengthening bones and muscles, it's so much more! Exercising as little as 30 minutes a day is enough to lower the risk factors for many diseases such as cardiovascular disease, type 2 diabetes, high blood pressure, and stroke.

When you exercise, it can even diminish the chance of some cancers that affect your stomach, esophagus, endometrium, bladder, breasts, lungs, colon, and kidneys. It can even improve recovery rates in people suffering from chronic diseases. It aids in lowering pain for those with arthritis, controls blood sugar, and gives independence of movement to people with disabilities.

At the end of the day, exercise increases your life because it combats various diseases, strengthens the body, so it can carry out its daily functions, and lowers the chances of falls in older people.

Yet it isn't just your body that sees the benefits. Your brain does as well. Exercise helps to lower short-term anxiety, improves learning capabilities and judgment skills, and improves your sleep. Overall, you should be exercising, whether you're fasting or not, there are just too many benefits to ignore.

EXERCISING WHILE FASTING

So, can you exercise while fasting? A bit of yes, and a bit of no. It all comes down to what fast you're trying, your diet, and what kind of exercise you want to do. The higher the intensity, the more difficult it'll be to get through a training session. Then there is the question as to when you should be training. Do you train before or after you eat?

While some people can train after eating, others prefer to work out on an empty stomach. When training on an empty stomach—especially after an overnight fast—you're forcing your body to get its energy from stored fat as there is little to no glucose available. Because of this, many people prefer to wake up, get a training session in, and then eat 2–3 hours later. Not only does this support the circadian rhythm, but it also allows for maximum HGH to be produced.

One of the key factors to training while fasting is remaining hydrated before, during, and after exercising. While fasting, you are already receiving less liquid as you aren't eating as frequently, but now you're adding training sessions, which will produce sweat. As you're losing more water and essential salts through sweating, you have to concentrate on replenishing them. Forgoing water will increase your fatigue, slow digestion, and cause bloat, headaches, thirst, and dry mouth. When you aren't sufficiently hydrated, your body cannot detox itself well, meaning your autophagy isn't running at its best. While you can attempt a dry fast, it's not recommended if you plan to exercise.

The type of training and its intensity will determine whether you need to eat before it or can complete it on an empty stomach. However, if you're new to fasting and exercise, it's a good idea to get used to one before adding the other. Changing your lifestyle too rapidly can result in more side effects than what the benefits are worth. When deciding to eat before a training session, do so 1–3 hours before, then only eat again two hours after finishing the exercise regimen. By waiting to have a meal after training you are encouraging protein synthesis to make new proteins.

Fasting Cardio

Attempting a cardio training session is possible during a fasting period as long as you are in good health and your fast isn't extended too long. When training on an empty stomach, there won't be any glucose reserves, meaning that endurance training (an hour or longer) may be difficult to achieve. In this state, exercising for too long can result in a person passing out. Endurance athletes may not be able to do cardio training without something to fuel them first.

When trying cardio training during a fasting period, start with 10 minutes of moderate exercise, followed by a small meal within a few hours. These sessions can slowly be built up to 30 minutes (possibly 40) but may require a small meal within half an hour of completion. Exercises you can try include cycling, the elliptical, jogging, or walking on an incline.

Exercising on an empty stomach allows for more fat burning than one that is fueled, which can cause exercise-induced nausea. However, an empty belly may make your performance tank, and you may struggle to build muscles. Stick to shorter sessions of training to prevent muscles from breaking down and increase the fat metabolism.

If you are a competitive athlete, you may have to adjust your fasting a few weeks before your event. This will ensure you have the right amount of glycogen in your muscles. Failure to do so could result in underperforming.

Fasting HIIT (High Intensity Interval Training)

Whether or not you can perform HIIT with or without a meal is dependent on your fitness level and how well adapted you are to your fasting technique. High-intensity interval training is where you use more calories in less time through spurts of energy at 85–90% of your maximum heart rate. The HIIT sessions shouldn't last longer than 30 minutes.

Most people, who aren't used to this form of exercise, may struggle to get through a training session without it being fueled. When in a fasted state, high-intensity training can cause low blood pressure, an abnormal heart rate, and all the side effects of low blood sugar.

You may also feel that you don't have the energy to complete the entire regimen. So, while fasting and HIIT can be combined—as it helps lower the body fat content—it'll be difficult, and you may find your performance lacking.

High-intensity interval training is best done when in a fed state—you'll need to eat 2–3 hours before training —allowing you to work out at the high intensity for longer. However, if you cannot move your fasting schedule to accommodate your training, you can include a small meal to fuel your training session. The exercise then uses up what you gave it, allowing you to continue your fast after the session.

Meal timing is vital when training at high intensities, as the food you eat is also used by the body to help recover from the session. Consider how your diet and fasting times should be adjusted to power a HIIT session.

Fasting Strength

Intermittent fasting doesn't promote muscle growth well, as strength exercises require glucose to fuel the muscles as they work. You are highly unlikely to bulk up—unless you have a specific diet—while lifting weights. Unless you're a bodybuilder, this is great for women, as intermittent fasting and strength training helps keep your muscles lean.

Doing strength training on an empty stomach will lead to lower endurance and performance and overeating after training, due to your body trying to compensate for what it has lost. If you prefer to do strength training, it's advised to have an easily digestible meal about two hours before your session. You will need a good source of protein—such as eggs—to get through your session. While the carbohydrates in your meal will power your muscles through the session, it's the protein that's broken down to help with muscle-protein synthesis. While training, your muscles go through muscle-protein breakdown. To recover from this, protein needs to be available to repair it.

Strength training is necessary for the body, it lowers insulin resistance and boosts HGH, leading to more fat burning. While not encouraged, if you want to strength train on an empty stomach, go for lighter weights and more repetitions. You should refuel with a high-protein meal soon after finishing your session to aid in the repair of muscles.

LISTEN TO YOUR BODY

Whichever training type you want to do is up to you, but realize at the end of the day that your body tells you if you can do it or not. Some people may feel on top of the world after exercise, while others feel like they've hit a wall. If you feel lightheaded, nauseous, or dizzy, you're pushing yourself too hard. Firstly, take a break, then reevaluate the intensity, when you're eating, and which fasting technique you're trying.

The 16:8 technique is one of the best techniques to couple with exercise as you can choose to train on an empty stomach or not. This also allows you to choose when you exercise and what kind of exercise to attempt.

In the beginning, only light to moderate exercise should be used in combination with short-term intermittent fasting and training. You'll need to concentrate on complex carbohydrates and proteins to fuel your body and aid in muscle recovery. Ensure you are replacing your electrolytes and hydrating well, as this will prevent many negative side effects during training.

You may find exercise while on an extended fast very difficult to do. This doesn't mean you have to give up on training. All you need to do is lower the intensity of your session and fuel it correctly.

Science is still on the fence as to whether you should fast and exercise at the same time. The most important part of combining the two is to ensure you listen to your body and stop before making yourself ill or getting injured.

SUCCESS STORY

Introducing Jennifer L. Scott, the creator of the channel *The Daily Connoisseur* on YouTube and a New York Times Best-Selling author of *Lessons from Madame Chic*. This 40-year-old mother of four set out to lose the baby fat she had picked up during pregnancy. However, there was a problem. She wasn't willing to count calories or cut any of her favorite meals. So, she turned to intermittent fasting.

Once educating herself about the different techniques available, she settled on using the 16:8 fasting technique. Within a year, not only did she lose the baby fat, but Jennifer is now sporting the same weight she had when she was in her 20s—116 pounds.

It wasn't an easy journey to begin, as she suffered from cravings during the evenings. However, after a year, she conquered fasting and it has now become her lifestyle. Realizing how easy it was to keep the weight off, Jennifer continues with her intermittent fasting.

Although she has lost the weight she set out to lose, she still enjoys the benefits of having high energy, no bloat, better mental clarity, and improved sleep. She finds that she's no longer ruled by food, and all the cravings for junk food are gone.

STARTING INTERMITTENT FASTING: TAKING CARE OF MUSCLE MASS WHILE INTERMITTENT FASTING

Because fasting can affect muscle mass, it's a good idea to protect it as much as possible. Although you don't want to bulk, you also don't want weakened muscles that can't carry you through the day. The best way to preserve your muscles is to be careful with how you train, the duration of your fast, and what you're eating.

When you start to exercise, it'll trigger the loss of fat and muscle. This is natural through the process of muscle-protein breakdown and muscle-protein synthesis. By eating protein, you absorb different kinds of amino acids that can be used to make new proteins and repair and strengthen muscles. However, while on a fast, you may not always have enough time to consume the protein required to handle growing muscles. Not only that, but growing muscles require more calories to be eaten. When trying to be deficient in calories, it will be difficult to grow muscles.

You will also need to consider the intensity and frequency at which you train, as this can affect how your muscles react. Strength training or moderate-intensity cardio (such as cycling or the elliptical) for 25–40 minutes three times a week won't cause your muscle mass to diminish. However, high intensities or longer sessions without proper protein refeed may. The best time to exercise is in the morning before breakfast or four hours before bed. However, this will depend on your fast and if you want to increase your muscle mass.

Exercise improves muscle cells' sensitivity to insulin, which is great because insulin resistance leads to poor absorption of amino acids. Meals with good quality complete proteins—not just BCAAs—are needed to help build and maintain muscles for training.

When concentrating on the 16:8 technique, you should limit yourself to two meals high in complete proteins. You will need at least 6–8 ounces of protein—more if you are bodybuilding—and each meal can be as high as 1,500 calories. Although this seems excessive, these calories are needed to grow the muscles and fuel your training sessions. Don't forget about the carbohydrates. Allow for about 50–70 grams of carbohydrates a day. This allows you to keep your insulin responses low, and allow your body to continue burning ketones as a fuel source.

Yet it isn't just protein that will keep your muscles in tip-top shape. When considering your diet, incorporate foods with calcium, vitamin B-complex, magnesium, vitamin D, and vitamin K. Without these nutrients you'll feel tired, be unable to complete training sessions, and lose muscle mass as your body tries to compensate.

Lastly, the fast you choose is vital, as it can affect how you build and preserve muscles. Prolonged fasting—72 or more hours—is too long and will result in your muscle mass diminishing when you try to exercise. This extended fast can lead to poor sleep, resulting in insomnia. This insomnia causes a cascading effect as cortisol starts to increase. Higher levels of cortisol prevent HGH from boosting metabolism and fat burning. Keep your fasts within the short-term range, or skip exercising during your long-term fasts to preserve your muscles.

So, should you exercise while you fast? A resounding yes! However, you may have to boost how much protein you eat. You can also supplement with creatine, BCAA, or protein supplements.

In the next chapter, we'll discuss the importance of meal preparation and scheduling your meals within your fast.

Wake up determined, go to bed satisfied.

— DWAYNE "THE ROCK" JOHNSON

feeling full for some time. Snacks such as popcorn (without the butter), raw vegetables, and low-sugar-content whole fruit are perfect. Avoid sauces for your food and salads, as they're empty calories and usually contain hidden sugars! Learn to cook with different herbs and spices. Not only does this save on calories, but some additions may help reduce feelings of hunger.

Lastly, you don't have to reach the pro or even advanced level if you don't want to. Push yourself to where you are comfortable and stay there. You can always challenge yourself with the occasional 24-hour fast if you'd like.

To help you along on your fasting journey, here is an eating plan for a week with the 16:8 fasting technique. It can easily be modified for the 18:6 technique too:

Monday

- Meal 1: Scrambled egg wrap with avocado.
- Snack 1: Small salad with greens, peppers, and tomatoes.
- Snack 2: Smoothie made with avocado, kale, and berries of choice.
- Meal 2: Stir fry with beef strips, cabbage, peppers, mushrooms, and onions.

Tuesday

- Meal 1: Whole-grain bread with tomatoes, hard boiled eggs, peppers, and feta cheese.
- Snack 1: A small banana with peanut butter or nut butter of choice.
- Snack 2: A portion of roasted chickpeas.
- Meal 2: Baked fish with asparagus on a bed of wild or brown rice.

Wednesday

- Meal 1: Hard boiled eggs with avocado, tomatoes, and chickpeas.
- Snack 1: Hummus with celery, cucumbers, and green beans.
- Snack 2: Greek yogurt with berries or granola.
- Meal 2: Quinoa with stir fry vegetables and a protein of your choice.

Thursday

- Meal 1: Omelet with feta, guacamole, peppers, and tomatoes.
- Snack 1: Apple slices with peanut butter or nut butter.
- Snack 2: A cup of berries with cottage cheese.

- Meal 2: Lentil curry with wild rice, cauliflower, green beans, and kale.

Friday

- Meal 1: Oats pancakes with peanut butter and banana slices dusted with cinnamon.
- Snack 1: A portion of trail mix.
- Snack 2: A few fat bombs.
- Meal 2: Roasted pork chops with steamed vegetables or salad.

Saturday

- Meal 1: A smoothie bowl with a choice of berries, nuts, and seeds.
- Snack 1: A cup of bone broth with a slice of whole-grain bread.
- Snack 2: Guacamole dip with seed crackers or sliced vegetables.
- Meal 2: Zoodles (zucchini noodles) with grilled chicken breasts with a choice of steamed vegetables.

Sunday

- Meal 1: Whole-grain toast with guacamole and a soft-boiled egg on steamed kale or fresh arugula.
- Snack 1: A portion of mixed nuts and seeds.
- Snack 2: Small chaffle with toppings of choice.
- Meal 2: Roasted vegetables, include some squashes, leafy vegetables, broccoli, and beets.

SUCCESS STORY

Artist and art model, Shannon Kringen, started the 16:8 fasting technique on July 5, 2018, to change how she looked. Although she had always been active, she struggled with her weight and a pronounced paunch that never seemed to disappear. Shannon had tried various diets and supplements, but nothing seemed to help keep the weight off.

Once she started fasting, not only did she see the physical changes but also mental changes. Within three months, she had dropped 25 pounds, the paunch was disappearing, and she found that her depression was improving. Although exercise had helped with her depression in the past, she found that intermittent fasting boosted the effects exercise gave her. Even her anxiety was starting to improve, and she finds that she's now able to cope easier when life throws curveballs at her.

As time progressed, and she found that she no longer suffered dizzy spells while fasting, she was able to push the duration of her fast. Now she can fast for about 20 hours with little to no side effects. When she's out and about, she always ensures she has some sort of meal with her, so she's never without food when she's meant to eat. Battling the bulge is difficult enough, but overcoming mental issues such as depression and anxiety is amazing! Because Shannon is feeling better, she has made fasting an integral part of her life.

STARTING INTERMITTENT FASTING: TAKING CARE OF PROTEIN REQUIREMENTS

Protein isn't just about building muscle; it also regulates your hunger. As it's so filling, it's difficult to eat the same quantity you used to during a shorter eating window. By consuming less protein, you can cause yourself to feel much hungrier than you should be. There needs to be a balance between how much protein you can eat while you can.

Protein comes from a variety of animal and plant sources, as well as supplements. You're spoiled for choice when it comes to choosing what you want to eat.

You'll need roughly 0.8 grams of protein to 2.2 pounds of your weight (Allarakha, 2021). Once you have worked out how much protein you need—it'll be in grams—you then divide what you need across your entire eating window.

Look at your eating schedule to see where you can supplement more protein into your diet. Why have a regular omelet when you can have an egg white omelet, which is higher in protein and just as filling? You can even exchange your guacamole dip for a cottage cheese dip. Consider other lean proteins such as chicken breast and tofu when making your favorite meals.

As a last resort, you can supplement protein through BCAA and protein drinks. With powdered-protein supplements, the range of meals you can add the supplement to increases. It can be added to smoothies, drinks, dusted over food, or even baked into pancakes or chaffles. Allow your imagination to run free, but be wary of the sugar content of some powdered-protein supplements. Consuming protein is easy when you look at everything that contains it. You don't need to stick to animal proteins. Explore the plant proteins to get the best of both worlds.

In the next chapter, we'll delve deeper into the therapeutic effects of fasting on the human body.

I've noticed when I fear something, if I just end up doing it, I'm grateful in the end.

— COLLEEN HOOVER

8

FASTING HEALS

E arlier, we touched on the healing benefits of fasting, and now we're going to go into detail. Fasting allows for a myriad of changes, one of which is stem cell regeneration. Although this field of study is in its infancy, it's showing interesting results. Looking at laboratory mice that fasted for 24 hours, it's noted that there was a reversal of age-related loss of intestinal stem cells (Trafton, 2018).

These stem cells are responsible for the maintenance of the intestinal lining, replacing it every five days. If any injury or infection occurs, these stem cells fix it. However, with age, these stem cells become less effective.

It's believed that when switching from glucose to fat metabolism, the stem cells start to regenerate, with an enhancement in their function. Despite this study using mice, it's a hint to what could await in human trials. If results are similar, fasting may be used to aid people with digestive tract infections and some cancers in the intestine. Yet, this is hardly the only way fasting can help people.

CANCER AND FASTING

Fasting isn't a cure for cancer, but it may be able to prevent the start and spread of the disease. One of the contributing factors to some cancers is obesity. When taking control of your weight, you're already taking a positive step to fight the disease.

Many animal studies, and some preliminary human studies, have shown that fasting can lower the risk of cancer as there is a decrease in cancer growth rates. Why is this? When fasting, there is lower blood glucose. Cancer cells require a lot of glucose to grow, and it's believed that when they're cut off from their energy source, they won't grow as readily. Autophagy causes the immune system to work better, allowing abnormal cells to be targeted and destroyed.

In a study by Di Biase et al. (2016), when mice models' fasting was combined with chemotherapy, it slowed the progress of skin and breast cancer. There was an increase in tumor-killing cells such as the common lymphoid progenitor cells (CLP) and tumor-infiltrating lymphocytes—a type of white blood cell. Together, these lymphocytes go into cancer cells and destroy them from the inside out. Although there are few human studies, those that have been done show that fasting causes a decrease in risk factors and biomarkers for cancer.

People on chemotherapy have stated that they feel better if they fasted before receiving the treatment. A likely reason for this is that by fasting, the cancer cells are more sensitive to chemotherapy, and the healthy cells are protected.

Many people make decisions based on animal models, but know that this only gives us a rough idea of what could happen in humans. It cannot be accepted as fact. Before it can definitely be said that cancer can be battled with fasting, it's a good idea to speak to your physician before incorporating fasting with other cancer treatment regimens.

PCOS AND FASTING

Polycystic ovary syndrome is a hormonal disorder that causes many symptoms such as weight gain, irregular or nonexistent periods, and fertility issues, just to name a few. Many sufferers of this disease are known to be insulin resistant, leading to struggles with blood sugar, high levels of insulin, and type 2 diabetes. A poor diet on top of PCOS will contribute further to weight and health issues.

One of the side effects of high insulin levels is that the body produces high levels of androgen—such as testosterone—in women. It's due to the abnormal levels of androgens that the ovaries develop poorly with a dip in reproductive health.

It's believed that with fasting, there'll be less glucose entering the body. Therefore, it doesn't need as much insulin to deal with it. With less insulin circulating, the cells become more sensitive to it, lowering the insulin resistance in the body. Less insulin will also improve ovarian function, decrease androgens, and increase fertility. Research is still new, but preliminary data is looking promising.

TYPE 2 DIABETES AND FASTING

Type 2 diabetes is caused by the body becoming more and more resistant to insulin's messages to accept glucose in the blood. With the cells not accepting the glucose, hyperglycemia, which is detrimental to the body, can occur as a result.

With fasting, the glucose levels are lower, and eventually, the cells lose their resistance to insulin. Fasting is known to cause not only a decrease in insulin resistance but also a decrease in post-meal sugar levels and fasting glucose levels. With enough time, type 2 diabetes can be reversed and kept in remission when continuing fasting and eating a well-balanced diet. That doesn't mean the disease will remain in remission if you continue to overeat, eat poorly, and not get some exercise. If you're worried about eating carbohydrates, cut out refined foods, and only eat whole foods. This way, you get enough fiber to control your blood sugar.

The one thing people living with type 2 diabetes need to be careful of is hypoglycemia. Hypoglycemia is when there isn't enough blood glucose. This often occurs in people who take medications or insulin to control their blood sugar. You should monitor your mood, blood sugar, and energy levels if you want to try fasting to avoid hypoglycemia. It may be necessary to have the support of a doctor—especially if you're on medication —and some friends to get you through the change you'll experience.

SUCCESS STORY

Melissa Bunch was a self-proclaimed food addict. It didn't matter if she was bored, anxious, stressed, or happy; she coped by eating food. As an emotional eater, her weight continued to yo-yo for 30 years. All this came to a head when she tragically had a miscarriage, and her blood pressure skyrocketed to 200/159, possibly resulting in a mini-stroke.

At 41 years old, she realized she needed to change her life, or there was a chance that she could die. After doing some research, she learned about intermittent fasting and hasn't looked back.

Within 10 months, she lost 100 pounds and managed to lower her blood pressure to a safer range. Fasting is who she is now, as it allows her to practice self-control when it comes to food. She still loves her meals but no longer indulges. Melissa can also enjoy her exercise more, as she is no longer carrying the extra 100 pounds she had in the past. To undergo a life-changing event and come out on top is commendable. This just proves all it takes is the right mindset to want to change for the better.

STARTING INTERMITTENT FASTING: TAKING CARE OF CARBS

There is no denying that carbohydrates cause a spike in blood sugar, and by eating less of them, there will be fewer insulin responses. Does this mean you should cut carbohydrates out of your diet? NO! Carbohydrates are one of the three macronutrients your body needs to function optimally.

A diet lower in carbohydrates does benefit people who want to get into ketosis faster, but completely cutting carbs out is a terrible idea. Most of the fiber your body needs comes from complex carbohydrates, and if you don't eat it, you'll suffer. Fiber not only keeps you regular but it slows down the digestion of carbohydrates and helps manage blood sugar, as glucose is released slower.

If trying a low-carb diet, you'll need to keep your carbohydrates at 20–60 grams per day. Combining this diet with intermittent fasting is possible but difficult as it comes with its own side effects known as keto flu.

Some symptoms include headaches, cramps, bad breath, and constipation. When going this route, take it slow. The 16:8 fasting technique is likely the best to try with a low-carb diet as there is less chance of you suffering severe deficiencies and side effects.

However, there is no need to be on a low-carb diet when fasting. You can aim for a lower-than-normal carbohydrate level and concentrate on complex carbs. Eat vegetables that grow above ground, as those that grow below ground tend to be higher in carbs. This includes potatoes, sweet potatoes, and carrots. You don't need to cut these out of your diet, but it's advised to eat starchy vegetables in moderation as they're calorie-dense.

Fruits may be difficult to incorporate into your diet when trying to keep your sugar levels down. After all, they developed their sweet taste to encourage the spread of their seeds. That doesn't mean you can't enjoy fruits. Berries, lemons, and avocado are all fruits you can enjoy, while other fruits should be eaten in moderation.

If you aren't prepared to eat a low-carb diet, you will need to monitor how many carbohydrates you are eating. Eating carbohydrates can affect your day—especially when eaten late at night, as it can keep you awake. Aim to eat the majority of your carbohydrates at the end of your fast while eating more protein closer to starting a fast.

In the next chapter, we'll take a deeper look at how the three macronutrients—fat, carbohydrates, and protein —influence the human body.

When you've seen beyond yourself, then you may find, peace of mind is waiting there.

— GEORGE HARRISON

9

THE NUTRIENTS YOU NEED
WHEN YOU'RE FASTING

E ven if you love eating food, this won't be impacted by fasting as there is no limit on what you can eat. If anything, fasting teaches you how to be mindful when eating. Food isn't just about filling your stomach and fueling you. Food is supposed to be pleasurable with its taste, smell, and texture. While fasting, you have less time to eat but more time to be creative with what you put on your plate.

Some foods don't fuel you as well as others, and though you can still enjoy some junk food now and again, it'll be more of an adventure to find foods that can replace it and be better. After all, chocolate isn't the only sweet treat that can satisfy your sweet tooth cravings.

Be creative, be colorful. Fasting is a process, not perfection. Eat what makes you feel happy and full through your fasting period. Play around with the food you love, and find new ones to fall in love with. Find creative ways to incorporate healthy fats, proteins, and carbohydrates in every meal you prepare and enjoy.

CARBOHYDRATES

Carbohydrates get a bad reputation from people that don't understand the macronutrient. Many people believe that carbs are pure sugar and are causing the rising obesity statistics. However, it's not carbohydrates that are causing people to get fat. The culprit is excessive eating and consuming refined carbs and sugar.

A regular diet should consist of 45–65% of carbohydrates, while a low-carb diet is 4–14%. This macronutrient is needed in the diet. It's in your best interest to have most of your carbohydrates come from plant sources, as they are high in energy, fiber, protein, minerals, vitamins, antioxidants, and phytonutrients.

Carbohydrates can be divided into two groups, complex and simple carbohydrates. Simple carbs are either mono- or disaccharides (one or two simple sugar molecules) and are found in foods such as milk, milk products, and fruit. These carbohydrates are easy to digest and will cause spikes of glucose which are followed by insulin. Complex carbohydrates are polysaccharides with many sugar molecules connected, and although this sounds worse for you, it's the opposite. Complex carbohydrates tend to be higher in fiber and are more difficult to digest. Whole grains, legumes, and vegetables are full of complex carbohydrates.

The problem with modern diets is that many carbohydrates have become refined. Grains are stripped of their bran and germ—which are rich in fiber—to give us white flour, rice, and bread. Fruits are stripped of their fiber to produce nothing more than sugar water. These refined carbohydrates, which are man-made, are one of the reasons obesity is as prevalent as it is. Without fiber, your body will digest the remaining carbohydrates quickly, leaving you feeling hungry a few short hours later.

Yet it isn't just refined sugars that play a role in the poor health of people today. It's their excessive consumption. Consume calories in excess long enough, and eventually, the weight starts to pack on.

The best way to avoid eating excess calories is to avoid all refined carbohydrates (or eat fewer of them) and expand your palate to enjoy more complex carbohydrates. The more fiber you eat with your food, the longer you'll feel full, and the slower the release of glucose will be. When eating from a 9-inch plate, ensure that at least half of it is full of fiber-rich vegetables.

PROTEIN

We've already discussed protein and its benefits to fasting. A diet with good protein sources can help boost metabolism, increase hormones that help reduce appetite (GLP-1, peptide YY, and cholecystokinin), and lower hormones that promote feelings of hunger—such as ghrelin. Because you feel full, you don't eat as much, leading to fewer calories being consumed. Protein also takes more energy to digest than other macronutrients. This combined with eating less food guarantees a calorie deficit. Eating protein with your last meal of the day also helps prevent late-night snacking and cravings.

However, can protein be bad for us? In a regular diet, protein should make up 10–35% of what we eat, but it can be easy to overeat this macronutrient due to the belief that eating more will cause weight loss. Except it won't. Per gram of protein, you get four calories, the same as with carbohydrates.

While some extra protein won't cause any harm, if increased too much, with a drop in carbohydrates, picking up weight will be the last of your worries. As with carbs, when too much protein is consumed, the body can only use so much before being forced to turn the excess into fat and excrete the remaining excess amino acids. Too much of anything is excess calories, regardless of what macronutrient you're eating.

One of the first signs of eating too much protein is the bad breath you can't get rid of. This is due to ketosis and can only be combated by drinking more water and brushing your teeth more frequently. If you have sacrificed carbohydrates for protein, you'll suffer from either constipation or diarrhea as you have no fiber to help regulate you.

Low-carb and high-protein diets tend to make people have low energy and become moody, as the gut bacteria no longer get the necessary fiber to thrive. Gut health is vital to your overall well-being, physically and mentally.

Excess protein produces excess nitrogen in the body, which needs to be flushed away. This can lead to dehydration if you're not replenishing your liquids frequently enough. Your kidneys will be working overtime to get rid of the excess nitrogen. This wouldn't be a problem with healthy kidneys, but with kidney problems, this can exacerbate the issues.

People who tend to overeat protein do so by eating too much red meat. Sure, it has protein, but it's also known to increase the risk factors of developing certain cancers and other chronic diseases. It isn't just red meat that's the culprit. When high amounts of red meat and full-fat dairy are consumed, this can lead to cardiovascular disease.

Eating excess amounts of protein—especially red meat—can result in lowered bone density. This is why it's important to have a diverse range of proteins, both from animal and plant sources.

It's important to remember that not all increased weight is because you're developing fat. With more protein, your muscles grow. This is why measuring inches is better than hopping onto a scale now and then.

FAT

Fat is the most controversial of all the macronutrients, and many people believe the myth that you should never eat fat. This is the worst thing you can do to your body. Without fat your organs aren't shielded, you can't generate energy from fatty acids (as they need to be consumed and can't be made by the body), certain hormones can't be made, and you can't absorb fat-soluble vitamins. You need fat, but the right fat or your health will suffer.

There are three types of fats: saturated fats, trans fats, and unsaturated fats. Trans fats are those you want to avoid as much as possible, as an adult shouldn't be consuming more than 5 grams a day. This type of fat can cause an increase in LDL cholesterol, which is considered by many as bad cholesterol, and lower the HDL. Although it can be found naturally in some meat and dairy, its artificial form is found in partially-hydrogenated vegetable oil. Trans fats are known to increase your risk of heart diseases, so avoid them as much as possible. Luckily, there has been a movement to remove this type of fat from foods.

Saturated fats are a little better for you, and as a woman, you can eat less than 20 grams per day. Many kinds of food include saturated fats such as palm oil, creams, meat, and meat products such as sausages. While this is a healthier option than trans fats, having too many saturated fats can also increase LDL cholesterol, resulting in heart disease and stroke. Saturated fats are found in avocado (in low levels), dark chocolate, fatty fish, and even processed foods such as desserts and baked goods.

The fat you want to concentrate on for your intermittent fasting has to be unsaturated fats. By eating this type of fat, you can control your cholesterol better. Unsaturated fats can be divided into mono- and polyunsaturated fats, of which the latter is very important. Polyunsaturated fats are the omega-3 and omega-6 fatty acids, which cannot be made by your body, so they need to be consumed. Monounsaturated fats are in avocados, most nuts and seeds, and some plant-based oils. Meanwhile, polyunsaturated fats are in plant-based oils such as soybean, sunflower seeds, and fish.

As a whole, unsaturated fats increase the HDL—or so-called "good" cholesterol—which helps remove the LDL to be taken to the liver and broken down. It's always better to have a higher HDL score than LDL.

Depending on what diet you're following, fat is generally acceptable at 10–35% of calories you consume. However, it's not just about quantity, it's about quality. One gram of fat gives you nine calories in return. Don't waste the calories on poor-quality fats that can increase your risk of cardiac disease and stroke. It's so easy to add good fats to your diet. It's as simple as adding an avocado to your salad or smoothie, having a portion of nuts as a snack, and eating fish at least twice a week.

Eating quality fats are great for your brain as it can lower inflammation. Yet, fat is great for the rest of your body too:

- It keeps you fuller for longer as it helps to regulate hormones that would increase your appetite.
- Food containing fat causes the stomach to empty slower, allowing you to feel fuller for longer.
- Fat carries the taste of what you're cooking, causing you to use less salt and sugar than needed.
- Some fat in your food helps with the health of your skin and hair.
- Fat is higher in energy than other macronutrients, and it can help keep your body burning fat when you lower the number of carbs you eat.

It's vital to remember that overeating any of the macronutrients will cause an increase in weight. Aim to keep within your calorie allowance, and you'll never have an excess, leading to increased weight.

SUCCESS STORY

Jen was always fit and healthy as a kid. She even managed to keep this up through college, but that changed one day. Her running coach insisted members of the track team be weighed in front of the rest of the team. This resulted in years of obsessive thoughts about weight.

Eventually, Jen met her husband, and together they had their first child in 2001. After the birth of her daughter, Jen was able to lose the baby weight and weighed 140–145 pounds, only about 10 pounds over what she was in college while running.

After some time, Jen and her husband started trying for a second child. Trying to get pregnant a second time was marred by many setbacks, but eventually, in 2005, her son was born. However, her weight didn't bounce back, and she gained 65 pounds. The obsessiveness with her weight surged, and Jen jumped onto every diet bandwagon there was to try and curb her increasing weight. During this time, she had become a stay-at-home mom.

In 2009, after unsuccessful attempts to lose weight, Jen turned to calorie counting and training for marathons. She was running 60–90 minutes every day, and counted calories obsessively, not allowing herself to enjoy any fun meals with her family. Within six months, she had dropped back to 126 pounds, but she couldn't enjoy her food as she once had.

She was able to continue this way of life for two years before she could no longer handle living with so many restrictions. From 2011 to 2021, she continued to live her life as normally as possible, even when Covid-19 hit the world. She had started working again but didn't feel great about how her body looked, so she hopped onto the scale to be met with a new weight of nearly 175 pounds. The weight gain rocked her self-image, and she realized she needed to do something to get back on track.

She discovered fasting and decided to try the 16:8 technique in combination with a low-carb diet. Within a few weeks, she had dropped 8 pounds effortlessly, and she wondered if this was a lifestyle she could continue.

She decided she could do better and switched to OMAD. Within four months, she had dropped a total of 46 pounds. Jen feels happier than she has in years. She feels healthy, her sleep has improved dramatically, and she no longer suffers from headaches that used to plague her life. Jen now effortlessly maintains her current weight and is living her best possible life, as she can have those occasional treats with her family if she wants to. Jen put a lot of work into her body, some good, some terrible, but in the end, with intermittent fasting, she achieved her health goals and is now happy.

STARTING INTERMITTENT FASTING: BENEFITS OF A PLANT-BASED DIET ON HUMAN GUT

Can you fast when you prefer to be on a plant-based diet? Of course! There are many benefits to being on a plant-based diet or substituting an animal-based meal for a plant-based one now and again. Not only is this healthier, but your guts will thank you.

In your intestines, there are trillions of microorganisms working together to ensure your health. Each type of microbe has its own unique function, and some can even make vitamins such as K, B2, and B9. However, many people fail to look after their gut microbes, leading to intestinal distress and even perforation of intestinal linings in severe cases. As you need to eat, so do these microbes, and the best way to do that is through fiber.

Fiber—a type of prebiotic—is the non-digestible part of whole foods, which travel through the stomach and end up in the intestines. Here it undergoes fermentation by the microbes as they feed. During their feeding, these microbes aid in the production of short-chain fatty acids (SCFA). Some of the fatty acids produced include butyrate, acetate, and propionate, all of which benefit your health by:

- regulating your metabolism
- lowering inflammation in the gut
- promoting insulin sensitivity
- helping with weight maintenance through feeling full
- improving immunity against pathogens
- upholding the integrity of the blood-brain barrier
- helping to regulate critical intestinal functions

As a plant-based diet is higher in fiber than an omnivorous diet, plant-based eaters tend to have more stable and diverse gut microbes. This can lead to them having a healthier lifestyle than others, but only if they get all the nutrients needed.

When trying plant-based meals, it's vital to remember that you must consume whole foods. Try to eat as little processed food as possible, as this can lead to gut inflammation and a change in microbe diversity. The diversity of the gut biome needs to be kept in the balance of the good microbes, as when the bad bacteria take over, you'll get ill.

You can add some probiotics (kefir, pickles, yogurt, etc.) to your diet. However, remember that not all of these will make it to your intestines as digestion will kill most of them. For this reason, a good combination of pre- and probiotics keeps the gut microbes happy.

So, the next time you have your third meal in a row with meat, consider how you would replace it with a protein and fiber-rich plant-based meal to get the optimum function from your gut microbes.

Now let's head onto the recipe section, so you can start planning your fasting around nutrient-dense, good meals.

We are not our best intentions. We are what we do.

— AMY DICKINSON

10

RECIPES

F asting can't be overcome without a plan, and that plan is to fill your feeding time with as many nutrient-dense meals within your eating window. Here are some examples to help you on your way. These are by no means the only recipes you can choose from. There are countless examples online for you to try; what is listed below is only a starting point.

SMOOTHIES

Smoothies are quick and easy, and you can combine vegetables and fruits in countless ways. Not a fan of cooked kale or spinach? Blend it into a smoothie to get the nutrients you need without forcing yourself to eat it from your plate.

Green Smoothie

If you're struggling to get your fiber in, give this smoothie by Intermittent Fasting for Vegans a try. Not only will it up your fiber content, but it's perfect for people who are lactose intolerant or practicing vegans.

Time: 5 minutes

Serving Size: 1 smoothie

Prep Time: 5 minutes

Cook Time: no cooking required

Nutritional Facts: for 1 smoothie

Calories: 550 kcal

Carbs: 114 g

Fat: 10 g

Protein: 12 g

Ingredients:

- 1 cup rice milk
- 5 dates, pitted
- 1 cup banana, sliced and frozen

- 1 cup pineapple, cubed and frozen
- ¼ cup raspberries, frozen
- 2 cups spinach
- 1 tbsp hemp seeds

Directions:

1. Add all the fruits to the blender and pulse blend until the fruit chunks are smaller. Scrape the side occasionally.
2. Slowly add the rice milk until you get the consistency you want. If you prefer an alternate plant-based milk product, then add that instead.
3. Pour into a glass and top with hemp seeds.
4. Enjoy immediately.

Orange and Cranberry Smoothie

Danielle has thrown together the perfect citrusy smoothie, high in vitamin C and fiber. Not only does this smoothie taste great, but it looks beautiful!

Time: 5 minutes

Serving Size: 1 smoothie

Prep Time: 5 minutes

Cook Time: no cooking required

Nutritional Facts: for 1 smoothie

Calories: 369 kcal

Carbs: 64.8 g

Fat: 1.6 g

Protein: 29.1 g

- 1 medium banana, sliced and frozen
- 1 navel orange, peeled and segmented
- 1 cup baby spinach or other greens
- 1 cup whole cranberries, frozen
- ¼ tsp cinnamon
- 0.7 oz vanilla protein powder, roughly 1 scoop
- additional liquid such as water or unsweetened almond, rice, or oats milk for blend

Directions:

1. Add the greens to the blender first, and then add all the other ingredients before blending.
2. Add any liquid to the mixture for your preferred consistency.
3. Serve immediately with a dusting of cinnamon.

Chunky Monkey Smoothie

Are you missing the sweet taste of chocolate? Why are you restricting yourself? Enjoy this chocolatey smoothie by Blair as a gentle way to break your fast.

Time: 5 minutes

Serving Size: 2 smoothies

Prep Time: 5 minutes

Cook Time: no cooking required

Nutritional Facts: ½ a serving size

Calories: 173 kcal

Carbs: 18 g

Fat: 6 g

Protein: 14 g

Ingredients:

- 1 banana, sliced and frozen
- 1-2 tbsp peanut butter
- 1 cup milk of choice
- 1-2 cups of ice
- 0.7 oz chocolate protein powder, usually 1 scoop
- 1 tbsp cocoa powder, unsweetened

- pinch of salt
- chocolate chips, for garnishing

Directions:

1. Add everything to the blender and blend until the mixture is smooth.
2. Split between two glasses and garnish with some chocolate chips.
3. Serve immediately.

BREAKFAST

Breakfast may not be the most important meal of the day for some, but for those who like to break your fast in the morning, this section is for you. And those who prefer to break their fast later in the day, who says breakfast meals need to be enjoyed when the sun comes up? Enjoy these tasty breakfast options whenever you make them.

PB&J Overnight Oats

Who doesn't love peanut butter and jelly? A portion of overnight oats is perfect for those who don't have time to make a nutritious breakfast in the morning. Luckily, The Editors of Women's Health have designed this easy breakfast which is as tasty as filling.

Time: 8 hours and 5 minutes

Serving Size: 1

Prep Time: 5 minutes

Cook Time: No cooking required, but should be left in the fridge for about eight hours.

Nutritional Facts: per serving

Calories: 455 kcal

Carbs: 36 g

Fat: 28 g

Protein: 20 g

Ingredients:

- ½ cup milk
- ¼ cup rolled oats, quick-cooking
- ¼ cup raspberries, mashed
- 3 tbsp raspberries, whole
- 3 tbsp peanut butter, creamy

Directions:

1. Add all the ingredients, except the whole raspberries, and mix well in a bowl.

2. If you like, scoop it into a mason jar, and store it sealed in the fridge for about eight hours.

3. When ready to eat, sprinkle the whole raspberries over the top and enjoy.

Lemon Blueberry Pancakes

Not only are pancakes delicious, but they can be eaten at any time of the day! There's no need to restrict this tasty meal, and thanks to Lacey Baier, you can make this recipe whenever the mood suits you.

Time: 20 minutes

Serving Size: 6 pancakes

Prep Time: 5 minutes

Cook Time: 15 minutes

Nutritional Facts: per pancake

Calories: 185 kcal

Carbs: 15.5 g

Fat: 7.1 g

Protein: 14.8 g

Ingredients:

- 3 egg whites
- ½ cup cottage cheese
- 2 tsp lemon juice, freshly squeezed
- ¼ cup water
- ½ cup rolled oats
- 1.4 oz vanilla protein powder, usually about 2 scoops
- ⅔ cup fresh blueberries, plus more for topping
- ¼ tsp lemon zest
- coconut oil, needed for greasing pan

Directions:

1. In a blender, add the egg whites, protein powder, cottage cheese, oats, lemon juice, and water.
2. Blend the mixture until smooth, occasionally stopping to scrape the sides of protein powder.
3. Pour the mixture into a bowl and gently fold in most of the blueberries.
4. Over medium heat, add a frying pan with some coconut oil to lightly coat it.
5. Once hot, add ⅓ of a cup of the mixture and cook for 2–4 minutes. The spatula should easily slide in under it.

6. Flip the pancake over and cook it for another 2–4 minutes. Check that the batter cooks all the way through.
7. Continue to cook pancakes until the batter is finished.
8. Enjoy the pancakes hot or allow them to cool.
9. Serve with a topping of blueberries, or other berries if you prefer.

SALADS

There is no need to spend a lot of time working over a hot stove when salads can be just as filling and satisfying as a cooked meal.

Cobb Salad

The cobb salad is high in good fats and proteins, with a side order of greens. Although many people have their unique twists to it, this salad comes from Barrett, and you won't be disappointed.

Time: 30 minutes

Serving Size: 6 servings

Prep Time: 20 minutes

Cook Time: 10 minutes

Nutritional Facts: per serving

Calories: 525 kcal

Carbs: 10.2 g

Fat: 39.9 g

Protein: 31.7 g

Ingredients:

- 3 eggs
- 3 cups chicken breast, cooked and chopped
- ¾ cup blue cheese, crumbled
- 6 slices bacon
- 2 tomatoes, chopped
- 1 avocado, peeled, pitted, and diced
- 1 head of lettuce, chopped
- 3 green onions, chopped
- Ranch-style salad dressing, optional

Directions:

1. Boil eggs for 3-5 minutes in a saucepan before removing from heat.
2. Allow eggs to rest in hot water for 10–12 minutes before peeling and chopping them.
3. While the eggs are cooling, cook the bacon in a skillet over medium heat for 7–10 minutes. Drain the bacon of excess fat and crumble it

before setting it aside.

4. Chop up the lettuce and divide it between four plates.

5. Add the remaining ingredients equally between the four plates before adding the cooled eggs and bacon.

6. Optionally, you can drizzle ranch sauce lightly over the salad.

7. If you don't like blue cheese, substitute your favorite cheese instead.

SOUPS

There is nothing better than a comforting cup of hot soup, regardless of the time of year. Many types of meat and vegetables can be used to make hearty soups. Experiment to find what you like best.

Three-Bean and Barley Soup

For this recipe by EatingWell Test Kitchen, you'll need a Dutch oven or a large pot for your stove. Not only is this soup packed full of fiber, but also full of flavor.

Time: 2 ½ hours

Serving Size: 6 servings

Prep Time: 5 minutes

Cook Time: 1 ¾–2 ½ hours

Nutritional Facts: 1 serving (1 ⅓ cups)

Calories: 205 kcal

Carbs: 36.4 g

Fat: 3.2 g

Protein: 8.8 g

Ingredients:

- 1 large carrot, diced
- 1 large onion, diced
- 1 large stalk celery, diced
- ½ cup pearl barley
- ⅓ cup dried great northern beans
- ⅓ cup dried black beans
- ⅓ cup dried kidney beans
- 4 cups of broth, chicken or vegetable
- 1 tbsp extra-virgin olive oil
- 9 cups water
- ½ tsp dried oregano
- 1 tbsp chili powder
- ¾ tsp salt
- 1 tsp ground cumin

Directions:

1. Add the oil to the Dutch oven or pot and set it to medium heat.
2. Add the carrots, onion, and celery and cook them until softened—this should take about five minutes.
3. Add the remaining ingredients and change the heat to high.
4. Wait for the mixture to simmer before reducing the heat to keep it simmering for the next 1 ½– 2 ½ hours, or until the beans are soft.
5. Occasionally check in to stir contents to prevent it from burning.
6. Once beans are soft, take 1 ⅓ cups and serve yourself a delicious soup.

SNACKS AND APPETIZERS

Snacks and appetizers are a great way to gently break a fast or a quick meal between your main meals. There's no need to weigh nut portions or prepare fresh hummus with these tasty treats.

Apple Almond Spice Muffins

Thanks to The Editors of Women's Health, we have this deliciously filling muffin that can either be a snack or breakfast, depending on what you want. Enjoy with some butter or fresh berries.

Time: 15 minutes

Serving Size: 10 muffins, 5 servings

Prep Time: 3 minutes

Cook Time: 12 minutes

Nutritional Facts: per serving

Calories: 484 kcal

Carbs: 16 g

Fat: 31 g

Protein: 40 g

Ingredients:

- 2 oz butter
- 4 large eggs
- 1 cup applesauce, unsweetened
- 2.8 oz vanilla protein powder, usually about 4 scoops
- 2 cups almond meal
- 2 tsp baking powder
- 1 tsp cloves
- 1 tsp allspice

- 1 tbsp cinnamon

Directions:

1. Preheat your oven to 350° F.
2. Prepare some muffin tins with nonstick spray and set them aside.
3. Add the butter to a bowl and microwave on low for 30 seconds.
4. Add all the dry ingredients into a large bowl and mix.
5. Add the wet ingredients to the bowl and mix until combined well.
6. Scoop the muffin mixture into the muffin tins until they are ¾ full.
7. Bake each tray of muffins for 12 minutes. Avoid overbaking, as this will make the muffins dry.
8. These muffins can be stored in airtight containers or frozen for later use.

No-Bake Carrot Cake Bars

Vegan treats don't need to be boring. Try this recipe by Kristen to satisfy your sweet tooth, and get all the nutrition you need to make it to that next main meal.

Time: 1 hour and 20 minutes

Serving Size: 8 bars

Prep Time: 20 minutes

Cook Time: No cooking required but needs to be frozen for an hour.

Nutritional Facts: 1 bar

Calories: 208 kcal

Carbs: 20 g

Fat: 12 g

Protein: 7 g

Ingredients:

- ½ cup carrots, cooked and mashed
- ¼ cup walnuts, chopped
- ¼ cup coconut flakes
- ¼ cup nut butter of choice
- 1 cup coconut flour
- 2 tbsp coconut oil, melted
- ¼ cup maple syrup
- ½ cup protein powder
- 2–6 tbsp coconut milk
- 1 teaspoon cinnamon
- ⅓ cup carrots, grated and chopped
- ⅛ teaspoon nutmeg
- a pinch of salt

Directions:

1. Whisk all the dry ingredients in a large bowl.
2. Pour in the liquid ingredients—but only about 2–3 tablespoons of coconut milk to start with— and mix until well combined.
3. If the mixture is too dry, slowly add the remaining coconut milk until the ingredients clump together.
4. Gently fold in the grated carrots, walnuts, and coconut flakes.
5. In an 8 x 8 baking pan, add parchment paper before adding the mixture.
6. Spread the mixture evenly and flatten.
7. Allow the mixture to rest in the freezer for an hour and then divide into eight equal pieces.
8. The pieces should remain in the fridge or freezer until eaten.

BREADS

Even when you're fasting, you get to enjoy bread. There are many types of bread to choose from online, which vary from savory to sweet.

Vegan Banana Bread

Banana bread is a treat most people struggle to give up, and now you don't have to, thanks to Carolyn!

Time: 2 hours and 20 minutes

Serving Size: 12 servings or 12 slices

Prep Time: 20 minutes

Cook Time: 1 hour cooking and 1 hour cooling

Nutritional Facts: 1 serving or per slice

Calories: 207 kcal

Carbs: 34.9 g

Fat: 7 g

Protein: 3.3 g

Ingredients:

- ¾ cup almond milk, unsweetened
- 5 tbsp water
- 1 ½ cups overripe bananas, mashed
- 2 cups white whole-wheat flour
- 2 tbsp flaxseed meal
- 2 tsp baking powder
- ½ tsp salt
- ¾ cup sugar

- 1 tsp vanilla extract
- ⅓ cup canola oil
- 1 tsp ground cinnamon
- ½ cup bittersweet chocolate chips (Optional)

Directions:

1. Preheat your oven to 350° F.
2. Use a nonstick spray on the inside of a 9 x 5-inch loaf pan.
3. In a small bowl, add the water and flaxseed meal and stir well. Allow to stand for a few minutes.
4. In a large bowl, add the vanilla essence, oil, almond milk, sugar, and the flaxseed mixture.
5. Mix in the mashed bananas until well combined.
6. Stir in the cinnamon, salt, baking powder, and flour.
7. Add the remaining wet ingredients until everything is well combined. If you want, add the chocolate chips and stir them in gently.
8. Slowly pour the batter into the pan and flatten the top.
9. Add the pan to the oven and cook for about an hour. Test the center by putting a toothpick in it. If it comes out clean, then it's done.

10. Let the banana bread remain in the pan for 10 minutes before adding it to a wire rack.
11. Allow the bread to cool for an hour before slicing.
12. At room temperature, the bread can last two days, but when frozen, it can last for about three months.

DESSERTS

A sweet tooth needs to be indulged, or dieting gets tricky. However, there are ways around the refined sugar treats we are so used to.

Fudge Brownies

Annie has come up with an amazing brownie recipe, perfect for the most stubborn of sweet lovers out there. Better yet? This recipe contains no refined sugar and is low in calories but full of fiber.

Time: 35 minutes

Serving Size: 9 servings

Prep Time: 5 minutes

Cook Time: 30 minutes

Nutritional Facts: per serving

Calories: 59 kcal

Carbs: 30 g

Fat: 1 g

Protein: 3 g

Ingredients:

- ¾ cup quick oats, gluten-free
- ¾ cup black beans, canned
- 1 tsp natural butter flavor
- ¼ cup water
- 7 oz yellow squash, cooked
- 1 tsp vanilla extract
- ¾ cup erythritol, granulated
- 1½ tsp baking powder
- ½ tsp liquid stevia
- ¼ cup cocoa powder, unsweetened
- ¼ tsp salt
- powdered erythritol, optional

Directions:

1. Preheat the oven to 350° F.
2. Using a nonstick cooking spray, coat the inside of an 8 x 8-inch pan and set it to one side.

3. Blend the oats in a blender and blend until it looks like flour.
4. Add the remaining ingredients to the blender and blend until a smooth consistency is reached.
5. Add the mixture to the pan and smooth the top before adding it to the oven.
6. Bake for 30 minutes, testing the center with a toothpick until it comes out clean.
7. Set brownies aside and allow them to cool—if you can wait that long.
8. Optionally, once cooled, dust the brownies with the powdered erythritol.

If you don't like the road you're walking, start paving another one!

— DOLLY PARTON

CONCLUSION

Fasting is an ancient technique deeply ingrained in our DNA. The hunter-gatherers of the past could skip meals now and again without detriment to their health, and so can you. By not eating for a set duration, your body is forced away from the glucose metabolism to fat metabolism. The longer you remain in a fasted state, the longer your body burns fat, improves autophagy, and the better you feel. Fasting isn't for everyone, and it's a good idea to ensure you aren't pregnant, have digestive issues, suffer from an eating disorder, or have a weak immune system before trying it.

There are many myths and fallacies surrounding fasting, which is why you should continue to research everything you read online before believing it. A well-known myth is that you shouldn't skip breakfast, when in actual fact, skipping breakfast won't ruin your day if you had a good meal the night before. Most people don't even eat breakfast, and they're doing fine.

There are several fasting techniques that you can try, from time-restricted fasts—16:8 or 18:6—to extended fasts such as alternate-day fasting. Fasting as a woman can be a little tricky, as our hormones play a big role in our weight loss journey. While men can handle the prolonged fasting periods, women tend not to. This is why you must experiment to see which fasting technique best suits you and your needs.

To have a successful fast, you need to fuel yourself well during your eating window, regardless of which fasting technique you want to try. Nutrient-dense foods containing quality proteins, healthy fats, and complex carbohydrates are the best fuel source your body can have when trying to fast.

You will feel hungry, and there is no way around that. You have trained your body to believe it needs food every 3–4 hours, and now it will demand it! During fasting, don't forget to hydrate yourself as drinks such as black coffee and tea, or water with some lemon juice, help curb hunger. However, it's important to listen to your body and not force yourself into a fast that can make you feel ill. Fasting is about building up to a goal.

Take your time and enjoy your journey; there's no reason to rush.

Exercise is possible when you fast, although the kind of exercise you do will determine when you should be training. Weight training is best suited for when you're in an eating window, while cardio and HIIT are possible during a fast. However, you may struggle with this training if you're not used to a combination of exercise and fasting. Again, ease into it.

Scheduling a fast and having a detailed plan of what you will eat is going to be your number one tool against hunger and failure. Start slow. Although a 16:8 fast is very popular, some people need more time to eat, so start at a 12:12 fast if you're struggling. If it's too easy, add a few extra hours to your fast until it starts feeling challenging.

Fasting isn't just about anecdotal evidence. There is science behind it. Many animal studies show great benefits to fasting, such as fighting cancer, reversing type 2 diabetes, easing PCOS, and regenerating stem cells in the intestine. Although animal studies don't give us the whole picture as of yet, preliminary human studies are starting to yield results that may be used by doctors in the future to combat many diseases.

That is fasting in a nutshell. We have covered several success stories of those who have traveled this road. People such as Jen, Melissa, and even Chris Pratt, all swear by intermittent fasting, which not only helped them lose weight but also changed their lives for the better. These people are just a fraction of the success stories out there. Are you prepared to become one of those success stories?

FINAL WORD FROM ME

Leaving a review on my book is incredibly important to me for several reasons. Firstly, as an author, I have put a lot of hard work and dedication into crafting my book. It is a reflection of my creativity, knowledge, and personal experience. Receiving feedback on my work validates my efforts and helps me improve as a writer. Reviews give me insights into what resonates with readers and what areas I can improve upon in my future works.

Secondly, leaving a review helps other potential readers make an informed decision about whether or not to read my book. As an avid reader myself, I know the value of honest and authentic reviews when deciding what book to invest my time and money in. A positive review can encourage others to pick up my book, while a critical review can help me understand where I need to make changes to improve the reading experience.

Lastly, reviews help me promote my book and increase its visibility in a highly competitive market. With millions of books available for readers to choose from, it can be challenging to stand out. Reviews help my book gain traction, and positive ones can even lead to features on bestseller lists or other promotional opportunities. In short, leaving a review is essential for readers to support and help authors succeed.

Thanks again for reading my book and the best of luck to you. May your success be as great as mine has been.

Christine xx

To leave a review from the United Kingdom (UK), please scan the QR code below:

To leave a review from the United States (US), please scan the QR code below:

REFERENCES

Abelsson, A. (2022, June 21). *Intermittent fasting and strength training: The ultimate guide.* StrengthLog. https://www.strengthlog.com/intermittent-fasting-and-strength-training/

Akram, M. (2022, January 10). *HIIT and intermittent fasting: Pros, cons & workout.* The Fitness Phantom. https://thefitnessphantom.com/hiit-and-intermittent-fasting

Alila Medical Media. (2019, August 5). *Intermittent fasting - how it works? Animation* [Video]. YouTube. https://www.youtube.com/watch?v=AhdFpWBeJSQ

Aliouche, H. (2022, January 22). *The effects of a plant-based diet on gut health.* News-Medical. https://www.news-medical.net/health/The-Effects-of-a-Plant-Based-Diet-on-Gut-Health.aspx

Allarakha, S. (2021, October 20). *How do you calculate how much protein you need a day?* MedicineNet. https://www.medicinenet.com/calculate_how_much_protein_you_need_a_day/article.htm

Animated biology With arpan. (2022, January 1). *Clinically proven benefits of intermittent fasting | intermittent fasting benefits | 5:2 technique* [Video]. YouTube. https://www.youtube.com/watch?v=EFphClArvO4

AshKals. (2017, April 14). Re: Intermittent fasting; success stories? *Reddit.* https://www.reddit.com/r/xxfitness/comments/658oti/intermittent_fasting_success_stories/

Atkins. (n.d.). *Intermittent fasting on a low carb diet: How it works.* https://www.atkins.com/how-it-works/intermittent-fasting

Aubrey, A., & Barclay, E. (2015, January 12). *Minifasting: How occasionally skipping meals may boost health.* Npr. https://www.npr.org/sections/thesalt/2015/01/12/376712920/minifasting-how-occasionally-skipping-meals-may-boost-health

Baier, L. (2018, April 26). *Lemon blueberry high protein pancakes.* A Sweet Pea Chef. https://www.asweetpeachef.com/lemon-blueberry-high-protein-pancakes/#wprm-recipe-container-20351

Baier, L. (2020, June 29). *How to break your fast: What to eat when you break your fast | intermittent fasting* [Video]. YouTube. https://www.youtube.com/watch?v=xzBy0RUQnuY

Baier, L. (2021, October 21). *Intermittent fasting meal plan | how to create your eating routine.* A Sweet Pea Chef. https://www.asweetpeachef.com/intermittent-fasting-meal-plan/

Bailey, E. (2021, November 30). *How the 5:2 intermittent fasting diet can help you lose weight.* Healthline. https://www.healthline.com/health-news/how-the-52-intermittent-fasting-diet-can-help-you-lose-weight

Barrett. (n.d.). *Cobb salad.* Allrecipes. https://www.allrecipes.com/recipe/14415/cobb-salad/

Barrow Neurological Institute. (n.d.). *About the pituitary gland.* https://www.barrowneuro.org/centers-programs/pituitary-and-neuroendocrine-disease/resources/about-the-pituitary-gland/

Benton, E., & Shiffer, E. (2022, February 11). *What is the warrior diet—and what do the reviews say about it?* Women's Health. https://www.womenshealthmag.com/weight-loss/a32329965/what-is-warrior-diet

Better Health Channel. (2012). *Obesity and hormones.* https://www.betterhealth.vic.gov.au/health/healthyliving/obesity-and-hormones

Biddulph, M. (2022, June 2). *Intermittent fasting 16:8: How-to, benefits and tips.* Live Science. https://www.livescience.com/intermittent-fasting-16-8

Bjarnadottir, A. (2018, May 31). *The beginner's guide to the 5:2 diet.* Healthline. https://www.healthline.com/nutrition/the-5-2-diet-guide

Bjarnadottir, A., & Kubala, J. (2020, August 4). *Alternate-Day fasting: A comprehensive beginner's guide.* Healthline. https://www.healthline.com/nutrition/alternate-day-fasting-guide

Blackwood, M. (2022, March 2). *18:6 intermittent fasting.* Healthier

Steps. https://healthiersteps.com/18-6-intermittent-fasting/

Blevins Primeau, A. S. (2018, December 28). *Intermittent fasting and cancer.* Cancer Therapy Advisor. https://www.cancertherapyadvisor.com/home/tools/fact-sheets/intermittent-fasting-and-cancer/

Boelen, A., Wiersinga, W. M., & Fliers, E. (2008). Fasting-Induced changes in the hypothalamus–pituitary–thyroid axis. *Thyroid,* 18(2), 123–129. https://doi.org/10.1089/thy.2007.0253

Booth, L. (n.d.). *Lifting weights while fasting: Should you do it?* Fitbod. https://fitbod.me/blog/lifting-weights-while-fasting/

Boyers, L. (2022, June 14). *What is circadian rhythm fasting & is it better than intermittent fasting?* MindBodyGreen. https://www.mindbodygreen.com/articles/what-is-circadian-rhythm-fasting/

Bradley, S., & Felbin, S. (2022, February 17). *10 intermittent fasting side effects that might mean it's not a great fit for you.* Women's Health. https://www.womenshealthmag.com/weight-loss/a29657614/intermittent-fasting-side-effects/

Brennan, D. (2021, October 25). *Psychological benefits of fasting.* WebMD. https://www.webmd.com/diet/psychological-benefits-of-fasting

Brick, S. (2021, May 20). *Alternate-Day fasting: Feast or famine for your health?* Greatist. https://greatist.com/health/alternate-day-fasting

Buckingham, C. (2022, April 19). *11 people who should never try intermittent fasting.* Eat This Not That. https://www.eatthis.com/is-intermittent-fasting-safe/

Bulletproof Staff. (2020, October 28). *Can you take supplements while fasting? What you need to know.* Bulletproof. https://www.bulletproof.com/supplements/dietary-supplements/supplements-while-fasting/

Bycott, B. (2019, October 22). *Does intermittent fasting work if you really love food?* Heated. https://heated.medium.com/intermittent-fasting-does-it-work-if-you-really-love-food-b383893bd4ab

Byrne, C. (2022, February 24). *Does protein make you gain weight? What you need to know.* Men's Health. https://www.menshealth.com/weight-loss/a39209663/does-protein-make-you-gain-weight/

Capritto, A. (2021, April 23). *What is the 5:2 diet?* Verywell Fit. https://www.verywellfit.com/5-2-diet-pros-cons-and-how-it-works-4770014

Casner, C. (2018, July). *Vegan banana bread.* EatingWell. https://www.eatingwell.com/recipe/266228/vegan-banana-bread/#recipe-body

Castaneda, R. (2022, May 27). *Intermittent fasting: Foods to eat and limit.* U.S. News & World Report. https://health.usnews.com/wellness/food/articles/intermittent-fasting-foods-to-eat-and-avoid

Centers for Disease Control and Prevention. (2022a, April 27). *Benefits of physical activity.* https://www.cdc.gov/physicalactivity/basics/pa-health/index.htm

Centers for Disease Control and Prevention. (2022b, June 3). *Losing weight.* https://www.cdc.gov/healthyweight/losing_weight/index.html

Chander, R. (2020, June 3). *I tried extreme fasting by eating once a day — here's what happened.* Healthline. https://www.healthline.com/health/food-nutrition/one-meal-a-day-diet

Charkalis, D. M. (2017, November 24). *Is this extreme form of intermittent fasting safe?* Prevention. https://www.prevention.com/weight-loss/a20507557/extended-fasting/

Cheung, C. (2022, June 14). *5 effective tips to gain muscle while intermittent fasting in 2022.* HealthCanal. https://www.healthcanal.com/life-style-fitness/intermittent-fasting-muscle-gain

chips15. (2017, April 14). *Re: Intermittent fasting; success stories?* Reddit. https://www.reddit.com/r/xxfitness/comments/658oti/intermittent_fasting_success_stories/

Cho, D. J. (2020, January 22). *Stars who've found success with intermittent fasting.* People. https://people.com/health/stars-who-do-intermittent-fasting/?slide=7010332#7010332

Cienfuegos, S., Corapi, S., Gabel, K., Ezpeleta, M., Kalam, F., Lin, S., Pavlou, V., & Varady, K. A. (2022). Effect of intermittent fasting on reproductive hormone levels in females and males: A review of human trials. *Nutrients, 14*(11), 2343. https://doi.org/10.3390/nu14112343

Clarke, N. (2019, August 2). *Why is it important to maintain a healthy body?* Livestrong. https://www.livestrong.com/article/416943-why-is-it-important-to-maintain-a-healthy-body/

Cleveland Clinic. (2020, July 21). *The best time of the day to eat carbs.* https://health.clevelandclinic.org/the-best-time-of-day-to-eat-carbs

Cleveland Clinic. (2022, April 4). *Pituitary gland.* https://my.cleveland clinic.org/health/body/21459-pituitary-gland

Clifton, K. K., Ma, C. X., Fontana, L., & Peterson, L. L. (2021). Intermittent fasting in the prevention and treatment of cancer. *CA: A Cancer Journal for Clinicians, 71*(6), 527–546. https://doi.org/10.3322/caac.21694

Clinical Dietetics Team. (2017, May 31). *Learn more about the effects of fasting on the body.* Cleveland Clinic Abu Dhabi. https://www.clevelandclinicabudhabi.ae/en/health-byte/pages/myths-and-facts-about-intermittent-fasting.aspx

Cole, W. (2018, May 31). *Intermittent fasting meal plan: Here's exactly when & what to eat.* MindBodyGreen. https://www.mindbodygreen.com/articles/intermittent-fasting-diet-plan-how-to-schedule-meals

Coppa, C. (2020, February 27). *10 mistakes you can make while intermittent fasting.* EatingWell. https://www.eatingwell.com/article/7676144/mistakes-you-can-make-while-intermittent-fasting/

Copper H2O. (2022). *Intermittent fasting and hydration: Complete guide (updated 2022).* Copper H2O. https://www.copperh2o.com/blogs/blog/the-complete-guide-to-intermittent-fasting-and-proper-hydration

Cronkleton, E. (2020, April 13). *Are there risks associated with eating too much protein?* Healthline. https://www.healthline.com/health/too-much-protein#risks

CTCA. (2021, June 9). *What you need to know about fasting and cancer.* Cancer Treatment Centers of America.

https://www.cancercenter.com/community/blog/2021/06/fasting-cancer

Danielle. (2021, September 24). *Orange cranberry greens protein smoothie.* Project Meal Plan.

https://projectmealplan.com/orange-cranberry-greens-protein-smoothie/#tasty-recipes-3099

DaVinci Healthcare Expert. (2019, June 21). *Does intermittent fasting boost human growth hormone (HGH) production?* DaVinci Laboratories. https://blog.davincilabs.com/blog/does-intermittent-fasting-boost-human-growth-hormone-hgh

Davis, N. (2021, July 14). *Benefits of fasted cardio: What happens when you work out on an empty stomach.* Healthline.

https://www.healthline.com/health/fitness/benefits-of-fasted-cardio

De Bellefonds, C. (2021, April 5). *4 sneaky ways protein is making you gain weight.* Women's Health.

https://www.womenshealthmag.com/weight-loss/a19992231/too-much-protein-0/

Di Biase, S., Lee, C., Brandhorst, S., Manes, B., Buono, R., Cheng, C.-W., Cacciottolo, M., Martin-Montalvo, A., de Cabo, R., Wei, M., Morgan, T. E., & Longo, V. D. (2016). Fasting-Mimicking diet reduces HO-1 to promote T cell-mediated tumor cytotoxicity. *Cancer Cell*, 30(1), 136–146. https://doi.org/10.1016/j.ccell.2016.06.005

Discovery Contributor. (2019, February 5). *The dangers of intermittent fasting.* Center for Discovery.

https://centerfordiscovery.com/blog/the-dangers-of-intermittent-fasting/

Dr. Eric Berg DC. (2019, December 9). *What really happens when we fast?* [Video]. YouTube. https://www.youtube.com/watch?v=vhmtoAYVRSo

Dr. Eric Berg DC. (2020, January 30). *Intermittent fasting and muscle mass gain – Dr.Berg* [Video]. YouTube. https://www.youtube.com/watch?v=DzknJGLYk9I

Dr. Mercola. (2012). *High-Intensity interval training and intermittent fasting - A winning combo for fat reduction and optimal fitness*. In Hoffman Centre for Integrative and Functional Medicine. https://hoffmancentre.com/wp-content/uploads/pdfs/exercise/ High_Intensity_Interval_Training.pdf

EatingWell Test Kitchen. (2016, April). *Southwestern three-bean & barley soup*. EatingWell. https://www.eatingwell.com/recipe/252788/ southwestern-three-bean-barley-soup/

Ederer, J. (2020, August 2). *What to drink while intermittent fasting*. Pique. https://blog.piquelife.com/what-to-drink-while-intermittent- fasting/

Ekberg, S. (2022, March 3). *What happens if you don't eat for 3 days?* [Video]. YouTube. https://www.youtube.com/watch?v=WOxg JE6QR2o&t=583s

Fertility Family. (2021, February 3). *How intermittent fasting can help with PCOS*. https://www.fertilityfamily.co.uk/blog/how-intermittent- fasting-can-help-with-pcos/

FitPro Team. (2020, October 23). *Intermittent fasting men vs. women*. FitPro Blog. https://www.fitpro.com/blog/intermittent-fasting- men-vs-women/

Forward. (2021, March 26). *Intermittent fasting 101: The science behind it, who it's good for and how to start*. https://goforward.com/blog/physi cal-health/intermittent-fasting-101-the-science-behind-it-who- its-good-for-and-how-to-start

Frank, G. (2016, September 14). *Why fat in your diet is good for weight loss, glowing skin and more*. Today. https://www.today.com/health/why-fat-your-diet-good-weight-loss- glowing-skin-t102800

Freire, T., Senior, A. M., Perks, R., Pulpitel, T., Clark, X., Brandon, A. E., Wahl, D., Hatchwell, L., Le Couteur, D. G., Cooney, G. J., Larance, M., Simpson, S. J., & Solon-Biet, S. M. (2020). Sex-specific meta- bolic responses to 6 hours of fasting during the active phase in young mice. *The Journal of Physiology*, 598(11), 2081–2092. https:// doi.org/10.1113/jp278806

Ganesan, K., Habboush, Y., & Sultan, S. (2018). Intermittent fasting:

The choice for a healthier lifestyle. *Cureus*, 10(7), e2947. https://doi. org/10.7759/cureus.2947

Gin Stephens, author and intermittent faster. (n.d.-a). *Jen T. from Michigan*. https://www.ginstephens.com/success-stories.html

Gin Stephens, author and intermittent faster. (n.d.-b). *Melissa Bunch*. https://www.ginstephens.com/success-stories.html

GMFH Editing Team. (2020, June 17). *Does a plant-based diet improve gut health? An interview with Hana Kahleova*. Gut Microbiota for Health. https://www.gutmicrobiotaforhealth.com/does-a-plant-based-diet-improve-gut-health-an-interview-with-hana-kahleova/

Griffith, T. (2018, September 29). *Fasting and cancer*. Healthline. https://www.healthline.com/health/fasting-and-cancer

Groth, L. (n.d.). *Chris Pratt is on the intermittent fasting train and wants you to join him*. LEAFtv. https://www.leaf.tv/13716281/chris-pratt-is-on-the-intermittent-fasting-train-and-wants-you-to-join-him/

Gunnars, K. (2017, May 29). *How protein can help you lose weight naturally*. Healthline. https://www.healthline.com/nutrition/how-protein-can-help-you-lose-weight

Gunnars, K. (2019, July 22). *11 myths about fasting and meal frequency*. Healthline. https://www.healthline.com/nutrition/11-myths-fasting-and-meal-frequency

Gunnars, K. (2021, May 13). *10 evidence-based health benefits of intermittent fasting*. Healthline. https://www.healthline.com/nutrition/10-health-benefits-of-intermittent-fasting

Gunnars, K. (2022, June 16). *Intermittent fasting 101 — the ultimate beginner's guide*. Healthline. https://www.healthline.com/nutrition/intermittent-fasting-guide#_noHeaderPrefixedContent

Hanka, S. (2021, July 2). *10 intermittent fasting benefits and potential risks*. Trifecta Nutrition. https://www.trifectanutrition.com/blog/intermittent-fasting-benefits-and-potential-risks

Harris, S. (2020, January 5). *What happens if you fast for a day?* Medical News Today. https://www.medicalnewstoday.com/articles/322065

Harvard Health Publishing. (2021, April 19). *Know the facts about fats*.

https://www.health.harvard.edu/staying-healthy/know-the-facts-about-fats

Harvard T.H. Chan. (2018, January 16). *Diet review: Intermittent fasting for weight loss.* https://www.hsph.harvard.edu/nutritionsource/healthy-weight/diet-reviews/intermittent-fasting

Heffernan, C. (2020, April 21). *Guest post: The history of intermittent fasting.* Physical Culture Study. https://physicalculturestudy.com/2020/04/21/guest-post-the-history-of-intermittent-fasting/

Heid, M. (2022, June 16). *The truth about fasting and type 2 diabetes.* Time. https://time.com/6188405/type-2-diabetes-intermittent-fasting

Heilbronn, L. K., Civitarese, A. E., Bogacka, I., Smith, S. R., Hulver, M., & Ravussin, E. (2005). Glucose tolerance and skeletal muscle gene expression in response to alternate day fasting. *Obesity Research,* 13(3), 574–581. https://doi.org/10.1038/oby.2005.61

Hoare, K. (2020, December 13). *Intermittent fasting and PCOS: What a nutritionist wants you to know.* Nutritionist Resource. https://www.nutritionist-resource.org.uk/blog/2020/12/13/intermittent-fasting-and-pcos-what-a-nutritionist-wants-you-to-know

Intermittent Fasting for Vegans. (n.d.). *Get your greens smoothie.* https://www.intermittentfastingforvegans.com/member-recipe/get-your-greens-smoothie/

ISSA. (2022, April 1). *Intermittent fasting: Women vs. men.* https://www.issaonline.com/blog/post/this-hot-diet-trend-is-not-recommended-for-women

Jennings, S. (2021, June 9). *"My health was off the rails and I knew it": How intermittent fasting changed everything.* The Courier-Journal. https://www.courier-journal.com/story/opinion/2021/06/09/intermittent-fasting-helped-me-lose-weight-improved-my-health/7596122002/

John Hopkins Medicine. (2021). *Intermittent fasting: What is it, and how does it work?* https://www.hopkinsmedicine.org/health/wellness-and-prevention/intermittent-fasting-what-is-it-and-how-does-it-work

Johns Hopkins Medicine. (2019). *Pituitary gland.* https://www.hopkins medicine.org/health/conditions-and-diseases/the-pituitary-gland

Johnson, J. (2019, January 28). *The 5:2 diet: A guide and meal plan.* Medical News Today. https://www.medicalnewstoday.com/arti cles/324303

Johnson, O. (2021, March 24). *Best foods to break a fast: Top 14 foods that make the fast to feast transition smooth.* BetterMe. https://betterme.world/articles/best-foods-to-break-a-fast/

Jrank. (n.d.). *Intermittent fasting.* https://reference.jrank.org/diets/ Intermittent_Fasting.html

Kandola, A. (2018, November 7). *Top 5 intermittent fasting benefits ranked.* Medical News Today. https://www.medicalnewstoday.com/ articles/323605

Kassel, G. (2021, June 17). *Should you be doing fasted cardio?* Shape. https://www.shape.com/fitness/tips/what-is-fasted-cardio-benefits

Kerndt, P. R., Naughton, J. L., Driscoll, C. E., & Loxterkamp, D. A. (1982). Fasting: The history, pathophysiology and complications. *The Western Journal of Medicine, 137,* 379–399. https://www.ncbi.nlm.nih.gov/pmc/articles/PMC1274154/pdf/west jmed00207-0055.pdf

Kubala, J. (2021, April 23). *9 potential intermittent fasting side effects.* Healthline. https://www.healthline.com/nutrition/intermittent-fasting-side-effects

Landes, E. (2022, January 26). *9 hormones that affect your weight — and how to improve them.* Healthline. https://www.healthline.com/nutrition/9-fixes-for-weight-hormones

Lawler, M. (2022a, February 10). *12 burning questions about intermittent fasting, answered.* Everyday Health. https://www.everydayhealth.com/diet-nutrition/burning-questions-about-intermittent-fasting-answered/

Lawler, M. (2022b, May 31). *12 possible health benefits of intermittent fasting.* Everyday Health. https://www.everydayhealth.com/diet-nutrition/possible-intermit tent-fasting-benefits/

Leal, D. (2021, September 13). *Does fasted cardio lead to greater weight loss?* Verywell Fit. https://www.verywellfit.com/is-fasted-cardio-really-better-for-fat-loss-4057205

Lean Squad. (2019a, March 13). *Intermittent fasting: How to curb your hunger.* https://lean-squad.com/blog/curb-hunger-if/

Lean Squad. (2019b, March 27). *Intermittent fasting: Morning workouts & breaking your fast.* https://lean-squad.com/blog/morning-workout-if/

Leffler, S. (2020, May 7). *Kourtney Kardashian shares her go-to intermittent fasting tips: Drink green tea, brush your teeth and more.* Us Weekly. https://www.usmagazine.com/food/pictures/intermittent-fasting-tips-from-kourtney-kardashian-pics/

Leiva, C. (2019, March 12). *9 tips for getting enough protein during intermittent fasting.* Insider. https://www.insider.com/getting-protein-while-fasting-2019-3

Leonard, J. (2020, January 17). *16:8 intermittent fasting: Benefits, how-to, and tips.* Medical News Today. https://www.medicalnewstoday.com/articles/327398#_noHeaderPrefixedContent

Leonard, J. (2020b, April 16). *7 ways to do intermittent fasting: Best methods and quick tips.* Medical News Today. https://www.medicalnewstoday.com/articles/322293

Lett, R. (2021a, September 8). *Guide to managing hunger, while intermittent fasting.* Span Health. https://www.span.health/blog/guide-to-hunger-while-intermittent-fasting

Lett, R. (2021b, September 8). *What to eat and drink while intermittent fasting.* Span Health. https://www.span.health/blog/what-to-eat-and-drink-while-intermittent-fasting

Lillien, L. (2020, December 16). *Do carbs make you gain weight?* Verywell Fit. https://www.verywellfit.com/do-carbs-make-you-gain-weight-4047400

Lindberg, S. (2020, September 1). *How to exercise safely during intermittent fasting.* Healthline. https://www.healthline.com/health/how-to-exercise-safely-intermittent-fasting

Link, R. (2021, March 22). *Can you drink water when fasting?* Healthline. https://www.healthline.com/nutrition/can-you-drink-water-when-fasting

Lite n' Easy. (2019, November 22). *7 benefits of meal planning.* https://www.liteneasy.com.au/7-benefits-of-meal-planning/

London, J. (2019, May 28). *What is the OMAD diet? What you need to know about this intermittent fasting weight-loss plan.* Good Housekeeping. https://www.goodhousekeeping.com/health/diet-nutrition/a27506052/omad-diet/

Lonergan, B. (2019, February 7). *Chunky monkey protein smoothie.* The Seasoned Mom. https://www.theseasonedmom.com/chunky-monkey-protein-smoothie/#recipe

Markowitz, A. (2017, January 16). *Vegan fudge brownies.* VegAnnie. https://www.vegannie.com/cake-bars-brownies/healthy-fudgy-brownies/

Martin, B., Golden, E., Carlson, O. D., Egan, J. M., Mattson, M. P., & Maudsley, S. (2008). Caloric restriction: Impact upon pituitary function and reproduction. *Ageing Research Reviews, 7*(3), 209–224. https://doi.org/10.1016/j.arr.2008.01.002

Matthews, M. (2020, December 23). *The risks and side effects of intermittent fasting you should know.* Men's Health. https://www.menshealth.com/health/a26052066/side-effects-of-intermittent-fasting/

Mazziotta, J. (2018, December 10). *Chris Pratt has already "lost a little weight" with intermittent fasting: "Works pretty good."* People. https://people.com/health/chris-pratt-intermittent-fasting-lost-weight/

McAuliffe, L. (2022, January 3). *The 20 hour fast: Benefits and how to.* Doctor Kiltz. https://www.doctorkiltz.com/20-hour-fast/

McKinnon, M. (2022, February 28). *Jennifer L. Scott's intermittent fasting success story.* Simple Nourished Living. https://simple-nourished-living.com/jennifer-scott-if-success/

Mdrive. (2022, February 8). *The guide to 18:6 intermittent fasting.* https://www.mdriveformen.com/blogs/the-driven/18-6-intermittent-fasting-schedule

MealPrep. (n.d.). *A guide to the 20:4 fast.* https://www.mealprep.com.au/intermittent-fasting/a-guide-to-the-204-fast/

Meola, K. (2019, November 22). *Kourtney Kardashian, Molly Sims, Hugh Jackman and other stars who swear by intermittent fasting.* Us Weekly. https://www.usmagazine.com/celebrity-body/pictures/intermit tent-fasting-diet-trend-celebrity-success-stories/ellie-goulding/

Metabolic Research Center. (n.d.). *Spontaneous meal skipping is an informal fasting protocol.* https://www.emetabolic.com/locations/ centers/cary/blog/weight-loss/spontaneous-meal-skipping-is-an-informal-fasting-protocol/

Midland, N. (2020, September 30). *18:6 intermittent fasting: Can eating only 2 full meals help you slim down?* BetterMe. https://betterme.world/articles/186-intermittent-fasting/

Migala, J. (2021, November 18). *OMAD diet: Is eating one meal a day safe and effective for weight loss?* Everyday Health. https://www.everydayhealth.com/diet-nutrition/omad-diet/

Migala, J. (2022, March 11). *The 7 types of intermittent fasting, and what to know about them.* Everyday Health. https://www.everydayhealth.com/diet-nutrition/diet/types-intermit tent-fasting-which-best-you/

Miroch52. (2017, April 14). Re: Intermittent fasting; success stories? *Reddit.* https://www.reddit.com/r/xxfitness/comments/658oti/ intermittent_fasting_success_stories/

MMA Fan. (2020, February 3). *What is the best form of intermittent fasting for cutting weight.* MMA Life. https://mmalife.com/whats-the-best-form-of-intermittent-fasting-for-weight-loss/

Morales-Brown, L. (2020, June 11). *Can you workout while doing an intermittent fast?* Medical News Today. https://www.medicalnewstoday.com/articles/intermittent-fasting-and-working-out

Mundi, M. (2022, May 5). *Is intermittent fasting good for you?* Mayo Clinic. https://www.mayoclinic.org/healthy-lifestyle/nutrition-and-healthy-eating/expert-answers/intermittent-fasting/faq-20441303

Nazario, B. (2004, April 23). *Another fat hormone may aid in weight loss.*

WebMD. https://www.webmd.com/diet/news/20040423/fat-hormone-weight-loss

Newsweek Amplify. (2020, October 18). *5 reasons why you should not try intermittent fasting.* Newsweek. https://www.newsweek.com/amplify/vegin-out-why-you-shouldnt-try-intermittent-fasting

NHS. (2022, February 23). *Facts about fat.* https://www.nhs.uk/live-well/eat-well/food-types/different-fats-nutrition

Nunez, K. (2020, February 18). *No-Bake carrot cake protein bars.* Clean Green Simple. https://cleangreensimple.com/recipe/no-bake-carrot-cake-protein-bars/

Olsen, K. (2019, October 11). *Why intermittent fasting is different for women.* Nutrafol. https://nutrafol.com/blog/intermittent-fasting-men-women/

Optimum Nutrition. (n.d.). *Intermittent fasting + protein: Combining strategies that may support weight management.* https://www.optimum nutrition.com/en-us/advice/nutrition/intermittent-fasting-and-protein

Osegueda, E. (2017, June 28). *Kourtney Kardashian shares details on her 24-hour fasting regimen and detox plan.* ET. https://www.etonline.com/news/220566_kourtney_kardashian_shares_details_on_her_24_hour_fasting_regimen_and_detox_plan

Pannell, N. (2018, August 27). *10 things you've heard about intermittent fasting that aren't true.* Insider. https://www.insider.com/intermittent-fasting-myths-2018-8

Panoff, L. (2019, September 26). *What breaks a fast? Foods, drinks, and supplements.* Healthline. https://www.healthline.com/nutrition/what-breaks-a-fast

Petrucci, K., & Flynn, P. (2017, April 10). *9 ways to stave off hunger when fasting.* Dummies. https://www.dummies.com/article/body-mind-spirit/physical-health-well-being/diet-nutrition/general-diet-nutrition/9-ways-to-stave-off-hunger-when-fasting-203866/

Preiato, D. (2019, May 23). *Everything you need to know about 48-hour fasting.* Healthline. https://www.healthline.com/nutrition/48-hour-fasting#_noHeaderPrefixedContent

Price, M., & Korman, J. (2020, August 25). *What you need to know about carbs & weight.* Priceless Nutrition & Wellness. https://www.price lessrd.com/blogposts/2020/8/25/what-you-need-to-know-about-carbs-amp-weight

Prospect Medical Systems. (n.d.). *Working out while intermittent fasting.* https://www.prospectmedical.com/resources/wellness-center/working-out-while-intermittent-fasting

Puckett, S. (2020, January 20). *Fasting for your health: What you need to know.* Boulder Medical Center. https://www.bouldermedicalcenter.com/6703-2/

Putka, S. (2021, July 9). *Male and female bodies can respond differently to intermittent fasting.* Inverse. https://www.inverse.com/mind-body/intermittent-fasting-difference-men-women

Rankin, J. (2022, June 17). *Alternate-day fasting: A beginner's guide.* Diet Doctor. https://www.dietdoctor.com/weight-loss/alternate-day-fasting

Revelant, J. (2021, October 28). *Is intermittent fasting safe for people with diabetes?* Everyday Health. https://www.everydayhealth.com/type-2-diabetes/diet/intermittent-fasting-safe-people-with-diabetes/

Rizzo, N. (2022, January 30). *What foods are best to eat on an intermittent fasting diet?* Greatist. https://greatist.com/eat/what-to-eat-on-an-intermittent-fasting-diet

Rogers, P. (2022, June 2). *Fasted weight training workouts.* Verywell Fit. https://www.verywellfit.com/weight-training-fat-loss-3969252

Ryan. (2021, August 10). *Intermittent fasting meal plan.* Ryan and Alex Duo Life. https://www.ryanandalex.com/intermittent-fasting-meal-plan/

Rynders, C. A., Thomas, E. A., Zaman, A., Pan, Z., Catenacci, V. A., & Melanson, E. L. (2019). Effectiveness of intermittent fasting and time-restricted feeding compared to continuous energy restriction for weight loss. *Nutrients*, 11(10), 2442. https://doi.org/10.3390/nu11102442

Schenkman, L. (2020, July 20). *The science behind intermittent fasting — and how you can make it work for you.* Ideas.Ted. https://ideas.ted.com/the-science-behind-intermittent-fasting-and-how-you-can-make-it-work-for-you/

Schwarz, N. A., Rigby, B. R., La Bounty, P., Shelmadine, B., & Bowden, R. G. (2011). A review of weight control strategies and their effects on the regulation of hormonal balance. *Journal of Nutrition and Metabolism*, 2011. https://doi.org/10.1155/2011/237932

Shemek, L. (2021, April). *Top 9 foods to eat while intermittent fasting according to a nutritionist.* iHerb. https://za.iherb.com/blog/best-intermittent-fasting-foods/1238

Shulman, S. (2018, August 31). *Here's what you should be eating while intermittent fasting to make the most of the diet.* Insider. https://www.insider.com/what-to-eat-while-intermittent-fasting-2018-8

Silver, N. (2019, March 29). *What happens if you don't eat for a day?* Healthline. https://www.healthline.com/health/food-nutrition/what-happens-if-you-dont-eat-for-a-day

Sinkus, T. (2022, May 3). *A complete guide to intermittent fasting + daily plan & schedule.* 21 Day Hero. https://21dayhero.com/intermittent-fasting-daily-plan/

Six Miles To Supper. (2018, October 17). *Intermittent fasting success story: Shannon Kringen* [Video]. YouTube. https://www.youtube.com/watch?v=cpudzfiuIEQ

Six Miles To Supper. (2020, October 3). *Karissa lost 125 pounds with intermittent fasting | success story | military wife | mom of two* [Video]. YouTube. https://www.youtube.com/watch?v=-KWDr3S-1v8

Smith, J. (n.d.). *The top intermittent fasting meal plan pdfs for 16/8, 20/4, 4:3, vegans, women, beginners and more with rules on what to eat, if coffee is OK and schedules to follow [part 1 of 2].* Eternal Oak. https://eternaloak.com/the-top-intermittent-fasting-meal-plan-pdfs-and-how-to-use-them/

Stanton, B. (2021, January 10). *Extended fasting: Benefits, tips, and how to*

get started. Keto-Mojo. https://keto-mojo.com/article/extended-fast
ing-benefits/

Streit, L., & Link, R. (2021, December 17). *What is 16/8 intermittent fast-ing? A beginner's guide.* Healthline.
https://www.healthline.com/nutrition/16-8-intermittent-fasting

Summer, J. (2022a, March 28). *Circadian rhythm fasting.* Sleep Founda-tion. https://www.sleepfoundation.org/nutrition/circadian-rhythm-fasting

Summer, J. (2022b, June 24). *Why intermittent fasting can lead to better sleep.* Sleep Foundation. https://www.sleepfoundation.org/physi
cal-health/intermittent-fasting-sleep

Tabalia, J. (2021, April 26). *Low-Carb intermittent fasting- everything you need to know.* BetterMe. https://betterme.world/articles/low-carb-intermittent-fasting/

The Editors of Women's Health. (2020, January 30). *Need an intermittent fasting meal plan? Here's your 7-day brunch and dinner plan to break your fast.* Women's Health. https://www.womenshealthmag.com/weight-loss/a30658778/intermittent-fasting-meal-plan-men-s-health/

The Lifestyle Dietitian. (n.d.). *PCOS and intermittent fasting.* https://
www.thelifestyledietitian.com.au/blog/2020/9/7/pcos-and-inter
mittent-fasting

Tinsley, G. (2017, December 3). *Does intermittent fasting make you gain or lose muscle?* Healthline.
https://www.healthline.com/nutrition/intermittent-fasting-muscle

Tomova, A., Bukovsky, I., Rembert, E., Yonas, W., Alwarith, J., Barnard, N. D., & Kahleova, H. (2019). The effects of vegetarian and vegan diets on gut microbiota. *Frontiers in Nutrition, 6*(47). https://doi.org/
10.3389/fnut.2019.00047

Trafton, A. (2018, May 3). *Fasting boosts stem cells' regenerative capacity.* Massachusetts Institute of Technology. https://news.mit.edu/2018/
fasting-boosts-stem-cells-regenerative-capacity-0503

Trumpfeller, G. (2020, July 22). *Everything you need to know about supple-ments and intermittent fasting.* Simple.
https://simple.life/blog/intermittent-fasting-and-supplements/

Vemuri, L. (2022, May 9). *What can you drink while fasting? Things you need to know in 2022.* HealthCanal.
https://www.healthcanal.com/life-style-fitness/what-can-you-drink-while-intermittent-fasting

Vetter, C. (2022, February 9). *What can you eat or drink when intermittent fasting, and what breaks a fast?* ZOE.
https://joinzoe.com/learn/what-to-eat-or-drink-while-intermittent-fasting

Vitti, A. (2021, November 2). *Intermittent fasting and hormonal health: What you need to know.* Flo Living. https://www.floliving.com/intermittent-fasting/

WebMD Editorial Contributors. (2021, April 8). *Is eating one meal a day safe?* WebMD. https://www.webmd.com/diet/is-eating-one-meal-a-day-safe

Weeks, C. (2020, February 27). *20 best foods to eat while intermittent fasting.* Eat This, Not That! https://www.eatthis.com/intermittent-fasting-diet-foods/

Werner, C. (2021, March 31). *Intermittent fasting and type 2 diabetes: Is it safe?* Healthline. https://www.healthline.com/health/type-2-diabetes/intermittent-fasting-and-diabetes-safe

Zelman, K. M. (2007, November). *The skinny on fat: Good fats vs. bad fats.* WebMD. https://www.webmd.com/diet/obesity/features/skinny-fat-good-fats-bad-fats

Zero. (2019, March 5). *Should you supplement while fasting?* https://www.zerofasting.com/should-you-supplement-while-fasting/

Printed in Great Britain
by Amazon

26733000R00136